THE
NEW
HIGH
INTENSITY
TRAINING

THE BEST MUSCLE-BUILDING SYSTEM
YOU'VE NEVER TRIED

THE
NEW
HIGH
INTENSITY
TRAINING

ELLINGTON DARDEN, PH.D.

RODALE

Printed in the United States of America
Rodale Inc. makes every effort to use acid-free ∞, recycled paper ♲.

Photography credits appear on page 239.

Book design by Carol Angstadt

Library of Congress Cataloging-in-Publication Data

Darden, Ellington, date.
    The new high-intensity training : the best muscle-building system you've never tried / Ellington Darden.
        p.   cm.
    Includes index.
    ISBN 1—59486—000—9 paperback
    1. Weight training.   2. Bodybuilding.   3. Muscle strength.   I. Title.
GV546.D29   2004
613.7'13—dc22   2004013394

Distributed to the trade by Holtzbrinck Publishers

2   4   6   8   10   9   7   5   3   1   paperback

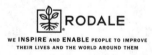

It's time to take charge
of your workouts by
having a challenging,
but realistic, plan.

CONTENTS

PART IV. Specialized HIT Routines

PART V. Body Transformation: A 6-Month HIT Course for Explosive Growth

PART VI. HIT Questions, Answers, and Trends

ACKNOWLEDGMENTS

I ACKNOWLEDGE AND thank the following people who made this project successful: Lou Schuler for editing the text as a seasoned insider, with just the right touch of magic; Jeanenne Darden, my wife, for adding readability and creativity to the initial manuscript; Mitch Mandel for photographing the illustrations with precision; Carol Angstadt for designing the book's interior with impact; and Karen Neely for keeping the entire publication on schedule.

Recognition extends to the individuals who experienced the "Old Days at Nautilus" and helped create the unique environment for HIT to evolve and thrive, primarily: Jim Flanagan, Ed Farnham, Kim Wood, Larry Gilmore, Dick Wall, Inge Cook, Casey Viator, Hector Hernandez, Scott LeGear, Pete Brown, Walt Anderson, Nick Orlando, Ken Hutchins, Brenda Hutchins, Tom Laputka, Roger Schwab, Dan Riley, Tom Grace, Wayne Westcott, Terry Carter, Bob Sikora, Dick Butkus, Eric Soderholm, Joe Cirulli, Terry Rogan, Gregg Webb, Gary Jones, Joe Mullen, Larry Evans, Terry Duschinski, Tim Patterson, Wes Brown, and Boyer Coe.

Special appreciation goes to Arthur Jones for being an exceptional friend, a master teacher, and a man of many adventures and much wisdom.

MORE THAN 90 carefully planned photos of Andy McCutcheon, a HIT martial artist and bodybuilder, are used throughout this book. Originally from Cambridge, England, he moved to Portland, Oregon, in 1992. During the photography, 38-year-old McCutcheon was in peak condition—at a body weight of 184 pounds, a height of 6 feet, and a fat level of 3.4 percent.

Get serious about achieving the muscular size that you've always wanted. Train now in the most efficient manner with the new HIT.

NEEDED NOW: ANOTHER REVOLUTION

THE FIRST REVOLUTION was started in 1970 by Arthur Jones. His ideas about high-intensity training—what we now call HIT—turned strength training and bodybuilding upside down. He invented Nautilus and MedX equipment. And, in the past decade, he had seemingly dropped off the face of the earth. Once a very public and very prolific man, Jones hadn't made an appearance or published an article since his retirement in 1996.

That's about the same time that my strength-training books, which helped explain and illustrate Jones's principles, went out of print. I hadn't written a serious training book since 1992. And unlike Jones, I didn't have the excuse of being retired.

All this came back to me when I visited Jones at his home in Ocala, Florida, on May 29, 2003. Jones still read an average of a book a day and perused dozens of magazines and research reports each week. And what he read had left him disgusted.

Everything he'd tried to change about strength training seemed forgotten. Where Jones had shown the benefits of shorter, more-intense, less-frequent workouts, magazines and books were once again promoting longer, less-intense, and more-frequent training. He was irritated and bitter. Who, he asked, was standing up and fighting for proper training?

The short answer: no one in the mainstream. At least, no one with Jones's tenacity. And certainly not me—I'd been on the sidelines for more than a decade.

Jones's anger that day was my wake-up call. My new mission was to bring high-intensity training back to the mainstream.

The Fun Is Gone

A month later, as I was outlining the chapters for this book, I got a call from my friend Chris Lund. Starting in the 1980s, Lund supplied the photography for some of my workout books, including *High-Intensity Bodybuilding* in 1984 and *BIG* in 1990. He's best-known for his work in *Muscle & Fitness* and *Flex,* Joe Weider's bodybuilding magazines, for which he's been a principal photographer for more than 20 years. Before that, he worked for Bob Kennedy's *MuscleMag International.* He's traveled the world, shooting all the major contests and all the greatest bodybuilders, year after year.

But this time, Lund had a confession. "You know, Ell, most of the fun's gone." For him, the good times ended after Dorian Yates won his second Mr. Olympia title, in 1993. The champions since then have been a different breed. "The drug use among these guys is horrendous—they're walking zombies. They're so out of it, it's almost impossible to be around them before the contests. And look what's happened to their bodies."

I had to agree. They'd gotten grotesquely big in their arms and legs, and their waistlines, swollen with massive doses of steroids and growth hormone, sometimes exceeded 40 inches.

That brought us, as it often does, to a familiar topic: the bodybuilders of the 1970s. "Casey Viator, Sergio Oliva, Arnold Schwarzenegger—those guys

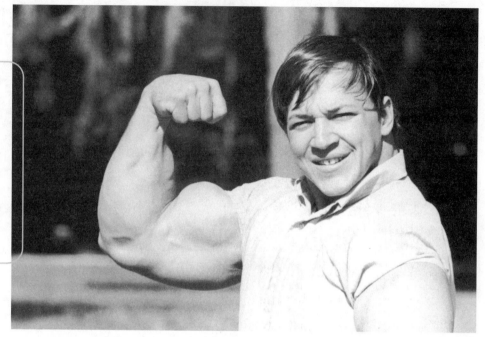

Casey Viator in 1971, at age 19, was the youngest-ever winner of the AAU Mr. America contest. You'll learn about Viator, and how Arthur Jones trained him, in parts I and IV.

were individuals; they had personalities," I said. Each one had a unique look. You could take their pictures, cut off the heads, and still tell which was which by the look of their muscles and the way they posed them.

"And you can throw in Mike Mentzer, Boyer Coe, Tom Platz, and Scott Wilson," Lund said.

The mention of Mentzer's name brought us back to Arthur Jones. Whereas the young bodybuilders today are into double-split routines, extended sets, and hour after hour of training, Mentzer was a Jones disciple, a high-intensity guy. Since Mentzer died in 2001, it seems, knowledge of high-intensity training, not to mention passion for it, has disappeared.

"Very few people understand it today," Lund said. "And it's a shame, a damn shame. Ell, you ought to get busy and do something about it."

Then I told him I was going to write a new HIT book. "Great! Great! Great!" he said. "The sooner the better."

High-Intensity Basics

In this book, I'm going to tell a lot of stories, for two reasons. First, of course, I like to tell them. I witnessed some significant moments in the history of strength training and bodybuilding, and I think you'll enjoy reading about them, just as I enjoy remembering them. Second, I think the stories I tell here make important points about training, and make them better than any textbook descriptions of exercise technique ever could.

In other words, it wasn't just what Jones taught that made HIT so important. It was *how* he taught it. Jones was unmatched at illustrating the fundamentals of training. I know this because for many years, Arthur Jones hammered the basics into me, a one-time Collegiate Mr. America and an aspiring

The Molecules of Muscle Growth

You might be surprised to know that a contracted biceps muscle, the approximate size of a tennis ball, is composed of more than 4.5 million units of growth material. Because muscle makes up about half of the average man's body weight, the total amounts of expansive matter throughout the muscular system number well into the billions.

That's right: Each of us has billions of units of growth potential in our muscles. But when a weight-trained muscle gets larger, what is it that actually grows? And, perhaps more important, how does it grow?

Muscle growth takes place at the microscopic, cellular level. The basic cells are called sarcomeres. Inside each sarcomere are strings of movement molecules called myosin, which, with tiny cross-bridges, connect to a thin protein filament called actin. Myosin, actin, and their interactions are salient to growth.

The key interaction must occur as a result of a muscular-system overload that causes the right amount of microtears and strains to the myosin and actin strings. When the strain on the muscle is focused and intense from multiple repetitions, the contractile mechanisms pull apart and tear slightly. This exposes frayed myosin and actin strands, which have the power to attract other growth elements. With adequate rest and nutrients, these units and elements are rewoven into thicker, stronger filaments with new branches.

Thus, the units of myosin and actin increase, which causes an expansion in the size of individual sarcomeres. Because the number of sarcomeres is set at birth, your only hope for muscle growth is to increase their size.

Progressing from micro to macro, the strings, or filaments, of myosin and actin form myofibrils, which are the threads running throughout the muscles. Groups of myofibrils bind together into individual sarcomeres or muscle fibers. Muscle fibers collect into bundles. The fiber bundles are then enclosed by a sheath of tissue, which provides specific muscles—such as the biceps, triceps, deltoids, and quadriceps—with their shape.

Regardless of a muscle's location, all growth from weight training must be stimulated by preparing and then tearing slightly at least some of the involved myosin and actin tissues. Without that slight tearing, they won't be receptive to developmental elements.

Got it? If not, please stop, go back, and reread the last paragraph.

That "preparing and then tearing slightly" is why *The New High-Intensity Training* is so effective. The HIT routines in this book, performed correctly, prepare and tear your exercised myosin and actin in just the right way. Too little tearing, and you won't get the muscle growth you want. Too much tearing, and you'll suffer injury, which could actually leave your muscles smaller.

The more advanced you become, the harder it is to get the proper amount of tearing. That's why this book shows you some advanced techniques: pre-exhaustion, reverse pre-exhaustion, breakdowns, forced repetitions, 1¼ repetitions, 1-minute repetitions, negative-only sets, negative-accentuated sets, and not-to-failure (NTF) training days.

Equally important, this course shows you how to plan your workout frequency to take advantage of your limited recovery ability. Applying the recommended long-term schedule supplies your body with proper rest. And that takes time. Only rest and time will allow your muscles to repair and rebuild themselves, and only fully recovered muscles will continue to respond and grow.

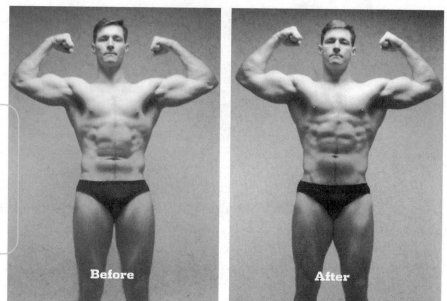

In only 2 weeks, David Hudlow built 18½ pounds of solid muscle and added 1⅜ inches on each upper arm. Part V describes the steps behind Hudlow's transformation.

Before

After

author of fitness books. This sound foundation prepared me to formulate the initial high-intensity training principles and guidelines that functioned, essentially, as the software for Jones's exercise equipment.

But that software clearly needs an upgrade. Lack of intensity, poor form, and excessive training are even *more* noticeable now among bodybuilders than they were in 1970, when Jones first revolutionized training.

And it's not just bodybuilders who can profit from HIT. If a guy is into heavy training today, chances are good he's *not* interested in becoming a professional bodybuilder. He simply wants to add solid, honest muscle to his body, without using anabolic steroids. Broad shoulders, powerful arms, a thick chest, muscular thighs, chiseled abs—these visions still keep him going. But he's not willing to spend half his adult life in a gym trying to achieve these goals. Efficiency and effectiveness are im-

portant to today's serious lifter. Or, at least, they should be.

What's needed is a renewal of the basics, the high-intensity principles that Jones launched. Once you understand these principles, there's even more: newer, more-scientific techniques that will increase the effectiveness of the basics.

This book provides a three-part foundation, followed by a three-part application.

Explosive Muscular Growth

Most of my books feature case studies of athletes who go through my programs. These subjects usually build 18 pounds of muscle in 6 weeks—gains the typical bodybuilder would kill for.

David Hudlow, who's featured in part V, did better than that. He gained 18½ pounds of muscle in just 2 weeks. That's an average of 1.32 pounds of muscle per day. I've never had anyone that I've personally trained build muscle that fast.

Over the next 4 months, he added another 23 pounds, which resulted in an overall gain of 41½ pounds. At the same time, he packed 2⅜ inches on each upper arm, 6 inches on his chest, and 3⅜ inches on each thigh. Any way you cut it, those are remarkable physical transformations.

What's the secret to such extraordinary growth?

It's applying both old and new high-intensity training concepts. These are concepts that, in many ways, are just the opposite of what most advanced lifters practice. For example, Hudlow got lean before he bulked up, instead of bulking up and then getting lean. He did whole-body routines instead of split workouts. He trained every other day, instead of daily. He did brief workouts instead of long ones, and he used strict form instead of cheating.

Furthermore, you need motivation and discipline to train in a manner that calls for demanding, challenging work. That's where Jones was unparalleled, both in his ideas and actions. I'll show you throughout this book how to apply his tips and techniques to your personal workouts. You'll get all the guidelines, practically applied, in part V. Exercise by exercise, workout by workout, week by week, month by month—you'll know precisely what to do, and perhaps more important, what not to do. You'll have the next-best thing to being personally directed and trained by me.

If you are tough enough to complete this course—and many trainees are not—even your mother will have a difficult time recognizing you with your more massive, muscular physique.

You'll look that different—GUARANTEED—after 6 months of the new HIT!

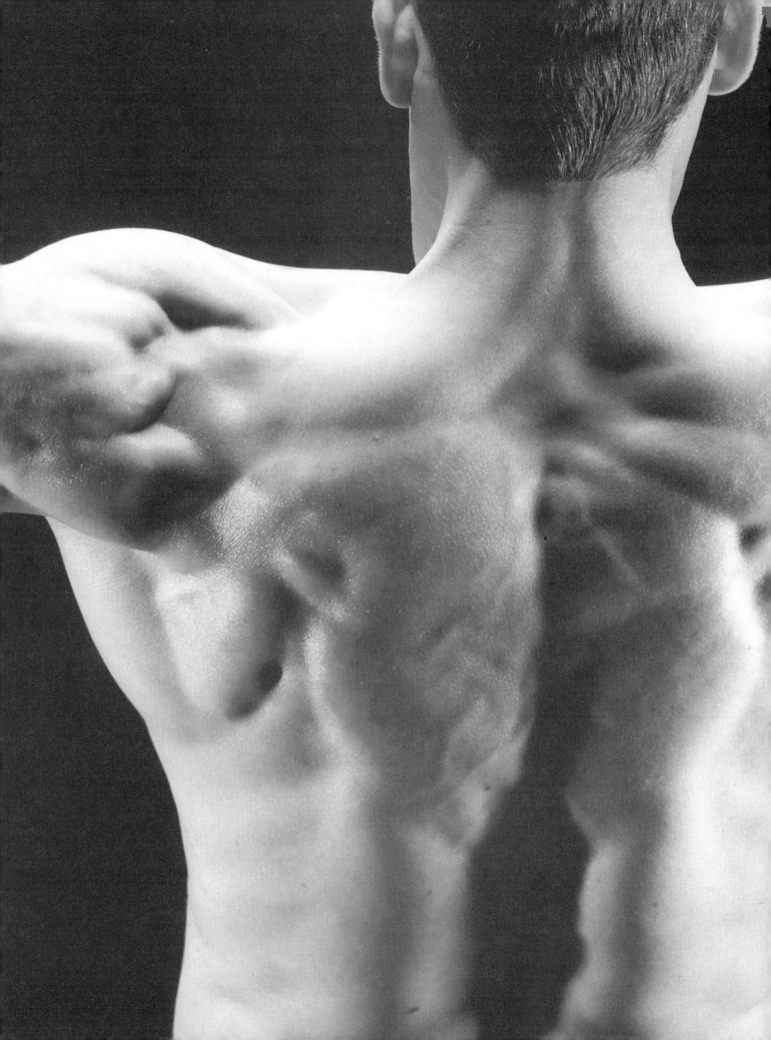

PART I

THE EMERGENCE OF HIGH-INTENSITY TRAINING

To infuse your body with renewed muscular growth, combine the best of HIT from the 1970s with the latest HIT techniques from 2004.

Chapter 1

THE ARTHUR JONES WAY

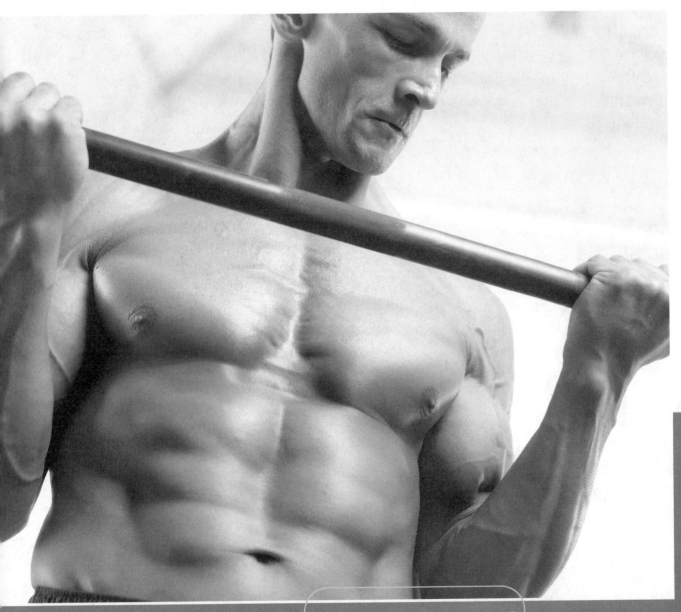

High-intensity exercise, performed the Arthur Jones way, requires attention to detail and unwavering determination. The muscle-stimulating results, however, are well worth the discipline.

"IF YOU'VE NEVER vomited from doing a set of barbell curls," Arthur Jones once said to me, "then you've never experienced outright hard work." *Outright hard work* was one of his descriptions of intensity, and to this day it's as good a definition as I've ever heard.

It was early in 1970, and I had been involved in weight training and bodybuilding for more than 10 years. But I had never vomited from a set of curls. I soon found out why.

Here's how Jones taught me to do it.

1. Load a barbell with a weight you can do for 10 repetitions in good form. Then decrease your weight by 10 pounds, because you probably over-estimated your strength.

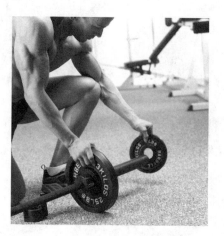

2. Grasp the bar with an underhand grip and stand erect.

3. Anchor your elbows firmly against the sides of your waist and keep them there.

4. Lean forward slightly, look down at your hands, and curl the bar smoothly and slowly. Don't move your head.

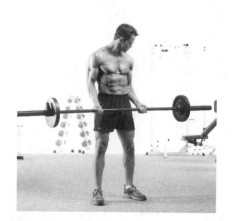

5. Pause briefly in the top position, but don't move your elbows forward. Keep your hands on the bar in front of your torso, as opposed to over your elbows.

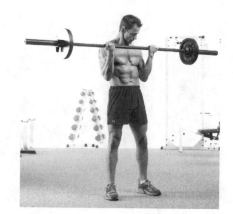

6. Lower the bar slowly and smoothly. Again, keep your elbows stable against your sides. The movement is very deliberate, and each repetition takes approximately 3 seconds going up and 3 seconds going down.

7. Repeat the curling movement using this exact form. You're aiming for 10 repetitions, but in reality, with this strict form, you hit the wall at 6.

8. Jones would now tell you to loosen your form slightly, by moving your elbows out and back-

ward and forward a little. You want to get the weight up, then focus on lowering it slowly. Sure enough, you get another repetition, but you can't get the next one. At this point, your biceps are very fatigued, and your forearms and hands are getting tired.

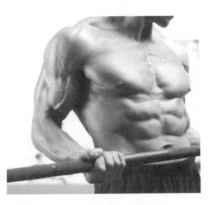

9. "Loosen your form even more," Jones would say, instructing you to lean forward and then backward while curling. Yep, you can do another, and, with Jones challenging you, you get one more— again concentrating on the negative, or lowering, phase. Those were repetitions 8 and 9. Now your lower back is killing you, your legs are shaking, your lungs are burning, and your heart rate is more than 180 beats per minute. Lucky for you, you've lost all feeling in your biceps, forearms, and hands.

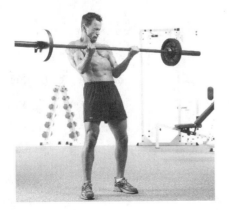

10. "Get one more repetition," Jones would inform you now. He'd be standing in front of you, telling you he'll help you get the last one. Slowly, the bar starts moving. You feel as if you're almost power-cleaning the barbell, using every muscle fiber to pull the weight to the top. When it gets there, Jones would give the final command.

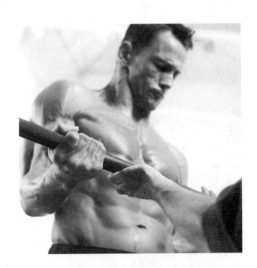

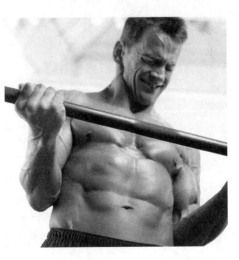

11. "Bring the bar halfway down and hold for a count of five. That's it—five, four, three, two, one! Now, ease the barbell to the floor."

Powerful Growth Stimulation

In something less than 1½ minutes, you've experienced *outright hard work* from one set of 10 repetitions of the barbell curl. Fifteen minutes later, if you can get off the floor, you'll still have a pump in your arms—and you'll feel much lighter without all that food in your stomach.

Now you understand why Jones often said, "If you *like* doing barbell curls, chances are you're doing them wrong."

By the end of the programs in this book, you'll be able to endure an entire workout of 12 exercises and perform each one just like those barbell curls I described. Your intensity will trigger maximum muscular-growth stimulation. And you'll understand why a high-intensity workout can't extend beyond those single sets of 12 exercises.

It took Arthur Jones 20 years to learn that two sets were better than four sets—and another 20 years to learn that one set was better than two sets. But he did learn. Most bodybuilders never grasp the concept.

The simple reason that one set is better than four sets is *intensity.* A more complete answer involves not only intensity but also the concepts of progression, form, duration, and frequency. The most comprehensive answer, which is necessary for a full understanding and application of all these concepts, is called achievement from generalization. Jones is truly, as much as any one word can describe a person, a generalist.

A Jones for Adventure

Jones first learned about generalization from being around medical doctors. They are highly edu-cated in a confined area, and he saw that their specialization leads to tunnel vision. A person with tunnel vision can rarely see more than a single point of view. Specialization, Jones reasoned, is best suited for insects, not people.

As a generalist, Jones has read extensively about many subjects, traveled the globe, met people, tried new endeavors, and conducted his life without being afraid of making mistakes. He wanted to experience the world broadly, as opposed to narrowly. And he has.

He has raced through the Serengeti and over the Outback, down the Congo and up the Amazon, out of Bogotá and into Singapore. He has met a few good people and a long list of very bad people. He is a motivated man who has lived a complex life in search of "faster airplanes, bigger crocodiles, and younger women."

And somehow, he found the time to become one of the most important forces in the drive to make strength training mainstream.

Jones's life has been so scattered and transient that many of his older friends didn't even realize he was the genius behind Nautilus exercise equipment. They thought of Jones as a headstrong individual who was always ready to explore another part of the world.

In fact, of the 450,000 words in Jones's unpublished autobiography (which he let me read in 2000), only about 5,000 are specifically devoted to exercise—which begs the question: What does all this have to do with high-intensity training?

"Just everything," Jones would reply. "Diversity allowed me to approach strength training from different perspectives than those preceding me. Diversity was a huge part of my success." If you want to understand the *why* behind high-intensity training, or HIT, then you have to delve into the life of Arthur Jones.

According to Jones, what you experience or learn in one area has application in all others. A big part of his unusual wisdom has been his ability to make these transitions, associations, and connections.

I've personally witnessed Jones generate these connections hundreds of times. Many of them, and the stories that surround them, are presented throughout this book. Each story packs a thought-provoking wallop.

So let's take a brief glimpse into the life of Arthur Jones.

The Runaway

Arthur Jones was born on November 22, 1926, in Morrilton, Arkansas, where his father, a physician, owned a small hospital. His mother was also a physician, as were six other members of his immediate family. Several years later, Jones's family moved to Seminole, Oklahoma, which was in the middle of a huge oil field. Such a boomtown provided not only a good practice for doctors but also a rough crowd of oil workers, gamblers, prostitutes, loan sharks, thieves, and gunslingers. Young Arthur grew up around an intriguing cast of characters, including doctors who frequently worked 20 hours a day. Both the adventuring spirit and the old American work ethic were a big part of Jones's early years.

He taught himself to read, and by age 5 he could comprehend both English and German newspapers.

His formal schooling was brief. He quit shortly after starting the 10th grade. Studying on his own, he became fluent in eight languages—which proved advantageous in his travels.

"I first tried to run away from home at age 8, had become rather successful at it by age 11, and was gone most of the time from 11 until I was 14," Jones recalled when I spoke with him at his home recently. "When I turned 15, I had visited every state in the union and parts of Mexico, Canada, and British Honduras."

Jones began training with a barbell when he was 12 years old. He was interested in gymnastics at the time and was particularly adept at chinning and dipping movements. Barbell curls and overhead presses made him even better at both activities.

In 1939, he started flying airplanes, and he maintained an accurate log of all his flights until 1967. By that time, he had recorded 14,090 flights, involving 17,393.6 hours of flying, in every state in the United States and in 56 foreign countries.

He joined the Navy in 1941, when he was 15. Though still officially too young for combat, he was admitted, after making possibly the highest score ever recorded on the entrance classification test. "I had a perfect score," Jones said, "except for the final question. Just as I got to it, and it was a difficult math problem, time expired. But a friend of mine, who was good at math, had taken the same test a day earlier. He told me the night before that the last question was a tough one and that out of five possible responses, he had chosen answer number 3. After the test, he rechecked everything, and the correct response was number 2. As I walked up to hand in my answer sheet, I quickly marked number 2—which, in fact, was the correct answer. So, in truth, my perfect score was tainted."

After World War II, Jones applied his fighting, flying, and traveling experiences to capturing exotic animals in Mexico and South America. He caught, crated, and transported snakes, jaguars, monkeys, lizards, caimans, parrots, and even tropical fish, sending them off to zoos, circuses, and reptile shows. Of course, Jones's favorite animals were the largest; he was fascinated by their strength, agility, and grace.

"An alligator," Jones said, "will always act instinctively and, therefore, cannot make a mistake. He'll always be right. He may seem to make mistakes, but that's only because he would be in a situation where nothing he does would make any difference. Take an animal like that and give him the capacity to think, and all you've done is add the ability to make a mistake where previously no such faculty existed."

In 1950, Jones sold some monkeys to Ray Olive, who was running an animal exhibit in San Marcos, Texas. The two men soon became partners and established a place in Slidell, Louisiana, called Reptile Jungle. They kept the business for the next 8 years.

And during those 8 years, Jones systematically exercised with his barbells, despite the long hours and strenuous work.

"While we were in Slidell," Olive told me, "something happened that made an impression on Arthur. One night, he was doing squats with a heavy barbell in his front room. Suddenly, he lost control, dropped it, and it went through the floor. That started him thinking of building a machine someday that would make squatting with resistance safer.

"Arthur was working out hard in those days, and he got his body weight up to 200 pounds. It was all muscle. In Mexico City one night, it turned unusually cold, and he had to buy a coat. We went all over town until we found a size 50, which finally fit his arms and shoulders."

Into Africa

In March 1956, Jones was walking out of a drugstore in Slidell when a paperback book caught his attention. *River of Eyes,* by Brian Dempster, was about crocodiles, a subject Jones knew a lot about. But this book was so full of inaccuracies and exaggerations that Jones couldn't get it out of his mind. The next 11 years of his life, in fact, were filled with crocodiles.

He flew to Africa that summer and explored it every way he could—by boat, by Land Rover, by helicopter, by plane, and, when all else failed, by foot. Jones traveled the length of the Nile and the Congo Rivers in a canoe—twice. He caught 189 crocodiles that exceeded 11 feet in length, the largest of which was 15 feet 2¼ inches long, 9 feet 3 inches around the belly, and 2,306 pounds. Furthermore, he relocated the reptile successfully to the California Alligator Farm near Los Angeles.

He filmed many of his adventures, producing and directing hundreds of documentaries in an 8-year stretch. He even had a TV show, *Wild Cargo,* which was popular throughout the central United States in the 1960s.

Wherever Jones established his headquarters for longer than a month, he usually built a crude exercise machine of some sort. "Over a 20-year period, I must have built three dozen of them," he said. "No

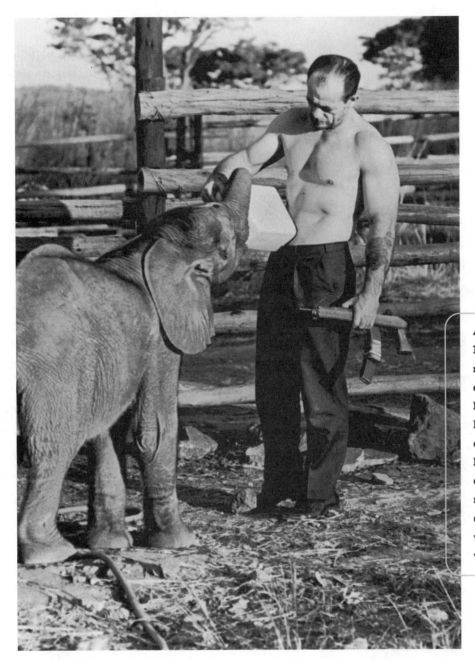

Arthur Jones, in early 1968, is shown feeding a malnourished baby elephant at his Rhodesian base camp. Notice also that Jones is carrying a lightweight M2 carbine, which was one of his primary means of protection during the African range wars that he had to cope with for many years.

two were exactly alike, but each one failed. They didn't fail to provide exercise, but they failed to satisfy me."

He was in Rhodesia (now Zimbabwe) in early 1968, when an important breakthrough occurred. "It was in the middle of the night, at 2:15 A.M., when I finally understood one of the major prob-

lems," he said. "We had been working on a pullover machine for the torso, and I suddenly realized that not only must the machine rotate on a common axis with the shoulders, but it also must *vary the resistance.* So I called an associate, carefully described what I wanted him to do, and told him to build it immediately and bring it to my house by 8:00 A.M. that same day. He did, and the new part was installed.

"When I got into the revised machine and moved back to the stretched position, it almost jerked my lats out by their roots. I didn't envision just how much the resistance had to change. So it, too, failed—but it failed so dramatically that I knew what would be required to make it work properly."

What Jones was talking about was the need to have variable resistance in an exercise machine— not just any variation in resistance, but resistance that varied according to the potential strength of the involved muscles. This was a major break-through.

The Natives Got Restless

After more than a decade in Africa, Jones had seen enough to fill a set of encyclopedias with pictures and stories. He had watched the unnecessary slaughter of thousands of elephants and what he felt was the stupidity behind it. He had filmed scenes littered with human bodies, devastated villages, and other atrocities wrought by bureaucrats and politicians.

It didn't take long for the government of Rhodesia to become increasingly uneasy with the man who had just built a new film studio and owned several automobiles and trucks, two airplanes, and a helicopter. Jones could no longer be ignored.

In 1968, Jones and his family left Rhodesia for a few days on business. They took with them only small suitcases with some personal belongings. When they returned, they found that everything had been confiscated, including more than $1.5 million worth of equipment.

Gone—and gone forever—were thousands of photographs and negatives, millions of feet of movie film, hundreds of books, papers, mementos, and rare collections.

Africa had cost Arthur Jones dearly. Besides losing all his possessions, including his last exercise machine, he had been bitten by poisonous snakes at least a dozen times, mauled by a lion, shot three times, and axed once. In addition, he'd crashed a jeep at 60 miles an hour and survived two plane crashes (which, for the record, weren't his fault).

But Africa had also given him an education that he'd later use to change the way many of us built our bodies. Flying small airplanes and helicopters taught him about physics, torque, and structural strength. Traveling with his life so often on the line made him a bold, dynamic leader. Moviemaking forced him to communicate quickly and effectively. Crocodiles enlightened him about basic instincts; elephants, about body mass and heat production; and lions, about the importance of intensity combined with rest.

On his return to the United States, he began the process that would eventually turn the bodybuilding world upside down.

Chapter 2

THE BLUE MONSTER
AND MASSIVE MUSCLES

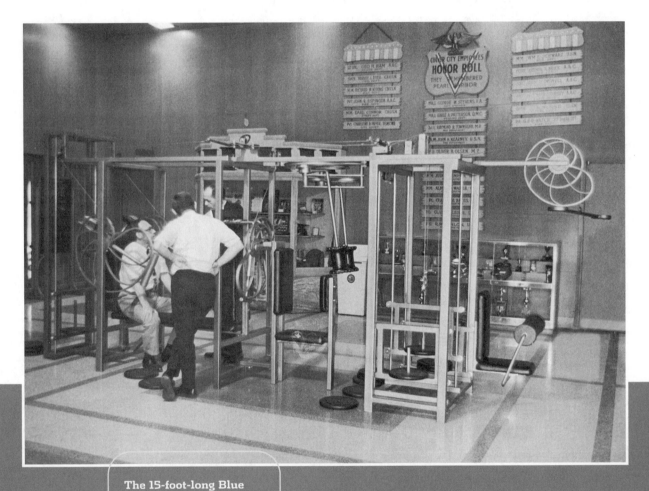

The 15-foot-long Blue Monster contained four unique machines that were painted blue. It received a lot of attention at the 1970 AAU Mr. America contest in Culver City, California.

JONES AND HIS family flew to Miami, Florida, in mid-1968. Jones still held out hope that he'd get his equipment back from the Rhodesian government, and he needed a business address to receive it. They rented a house in a small town called Lake Helen, near DeLand, in central Florida.

While waiting on word from Rhodesia (which would never come), Jones decided to start training again with weights. Naturally, he began tinkering with rebuilding, and improving, some of his previous machines. His nephew, Scott LeGear, joined in with the training and tinkering. They exercised primarily in Jones's living room.

"There was a chinning bar bolted to the staircase," LeGear recalled. "There was a bench with racks and a barbell in the middle of the living room, with weights scattered all around. We performed all the basic exercises: chinups, presses, curls, squats, and stiff-legged deadlifts.

"Eventually, we started thinking, 'What if we do this?' or 'What if we do that?' That was when we started going over to Sarge's place. Sarge had a shop called DeLand Metal Craft. He made wrought-iron railings and did general metal jobs. For us, the place became an after-hours work facility.

"The first thing we built was a curling machine. It was really crude. We'd haul it over to Arthur's front porch, try it for a few workouts, haul it back to the shop, rework some of it, haul it back, and try it again. That type of thing went on for weeks. More than anything, we started figuring out what we did *not* want. So we were that much closer to what we did want.

"Then we started into something Arthur had been trying to solve for 20 years: how best to work the lats," LeGear said. "You can't completely work the latissimus dorsi with a chinning bar or barbell, because the arms and hands get tired first. Arthur conceived the idea of bypassing the hands and using a pad against the upper arms. That was the beginning of a radical departure from the barbell. We were thinking, 'What are we really doing here? We're not lifting barbells.' Suddenly came the realization that barbells are no more than a tool to perform a function. 'Identify the function,' we decided, 'and maybe we can make a better tool.'

"Most of the conceptual developments of the single-joint, rotary machines materialized during that period. Arthur, I think, had never taken the time to concentrate on the science of exercise. He had plenty of time in 1968—we both did."

A Different Take on Bodybuilding

Jones always trained brutally hard, and he kept precise records of everything that he did, exercise by exercise, repetition by repetition, which included measurements and body weight. He rapidly increased his muscular size and strength in 1969, as he always did with training. But this time, he literally had nothing to do but train and think about training, which is why he decided to write about it for the first time. He outlined his workouts in an article and sent it to the prominent bodybuilding magazines of the time.

First, he tried Bob Hoffman and *Strength and Health* magazine. He waited and waited but got no response. Then he sent the material to Joe Weider at *Muscle Builder/Power* magazine. Again, no response.

Finally, in disgust, he reworked the piece into an attack on, and insult to, just about everyone connected to bodybuilding. "Quit emulating the workouts of the men who are winning the titles," he proclaimed. "Most of them can't even spell the word *muscle.*" He then introduced his training formula: "If you want to get bigger and stronger, you must make measurable, stair-step progress during each workout. Size always precedes strength. If you're not making gains workout by workout, your exercise intensity is too low. The key is to train harder, to continue each exercise until no additional repetitions are possible. But if you train harder, you must train less."

I can't emphasize enough how radical these ideas were. The dominant muscle-building philosophy of the 1960s, advanced in all the bodybuilding magazines, was that *more exercise is better.* To be successful, you had to blitz and bomb all your major muscle groups with angle training, multiple sets, and double-split routines. It wasn't unusual for a young bodybuilder to spend 3 to 4 hours a day in a gym, 6 days per week.

This time, Jones sent the article to Peary Rader of *IronMan* magazine, but he didn't expect anything to happen. He figured Rader would ignore him, just as the others had, and admitted to himself that he'd written the pages more for his own satisfaction than for any public airing of his views. Writing it all down simply made him feel better.

Rader, however, thought the piece was eye-opening. He called Jones immediately, and they talked at length. By the end of the conversation, Jones had agreed to do a series of articles for *IronMan,* which started in the spring of 1970 and continued for the next 4 years.

Rise of the Machines

Jones had spent 20 years building and rebuilding exercise machines but never with any intention of getting into the business of making and selling them. He also didn't mind using his machines, crude as they were, to demonstrate the shortcomings of various barbell and dumbbell exercises. He included photos of two of them in one of his articles, expecting nothing beyond a uniformly angry response from *IronMan*'s readers. Who wants to be told that everything they'd believed for years, if not decades, was wrong?

Instead, he received letters almost daily from readers who wanted to know more about the machines he was talking about. At that time, the two he'd photographed were the only ones he'd actually built. (He kept them on his back porch in Lake Helen.) His articles, though, described several others, which at that time existed only in his head.

The letters kept coming, and some readers even sent money as deposits toward the purchase of his machines. So Jones decided to test their commercial potential by showing some examples at the next AAU (Amateur Athletic Union) Mr. America contest, which was scheduled for mid-June 1970 in Los Angeles. He had just 3 months to build a prototype machine, and his nephew had already departed to study photography.

He knew he needed help, and the only guy he could think of to recruit was a weight lifter with whom he'd gotten into an argument in a parking lot several months before. He didn't even know the man's name. But, with a few queries, he learned that his prospective accomplice was Larry Gilmore, a competitive lifter and employee of the local telephone company.

Jones and Gilmore quickly established an enduring friendship. With Gilmore handling the welding and fabricating, the two worked nights and weekends to create Jones's prototype machine.

What emerged was the Blue Monster: a combination of four machines, all connected in a 15-foot-long apparatus and painted blue. Jones didn't particularly like the configuration, but he knew that displaying a big machine—perhaps the biggest one ever—would make a stronger first impression.

Jones hauled it to Los Angeles personally in a rented trailer. Sure enough, the Blue Monster was the talk of the show. Once you saw it, it was impossible to forget.

I know, because I was there. I walked by the Blue Monster in the lobby on the first day, stopped and did a double take, but didn't try it. I tried several stations on the second day, but I didn't get a chance to talk with Jones.

After the competition, I sat next to an AAU official, Karo Whitfield, on the flight from Los Angeles back to Atlanta. "I've seen it all in my 50 years in the bodybuilding business," said Whitfield, who was about 70 at the time. "But this machine and the man behind it are clearly different. Don't be surprised if Jones turns the business upside down."

My Background

So now that I've put myself in the story, let me tell you a little more about my background. I grew up in Conroe, Texas, and began lifting weights in 1959, when I was in the ninth grade. I started entering physique contests seriously in 1964, while I was an undergraduate at Baylor University. I competed in my first national event in 1967, the Junior Mr. USA, and placed fifth.

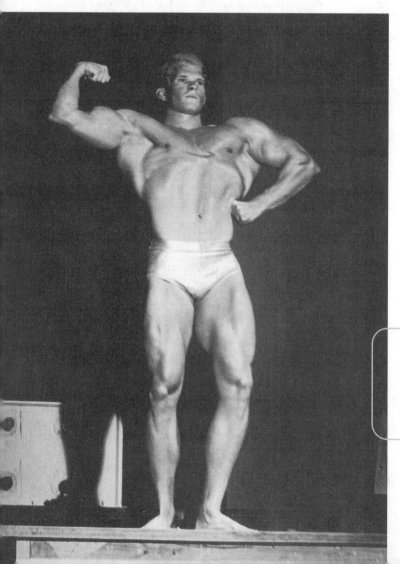

I grew up in Conroe, Texas, and won the 1969 Mr. Texas contest. As an interesting side note, Casey Viator, at age 17 and weighing 175 pounds, finished in fourth place.

In 1969, I won the Mr. Texas title and placed 10th in the AAU Mr. America contest, which Boyer Coe won. (Coe was from Lafayette, Louisiana, and we met in 1965, when he won Mr. Texas.)

At the time of the 1970 Mr. America, I was in graduate school at Florida State University in Tallahassee. My typical training consisted of split routines of 10 to 15 exercises performed for three to five sets. I usually trained 4 or 5 days a week, with each workout lasting at least 90 minutes. Most of the competitors in the national events performed similar routines.

I finished out of the top 10 at the 1970 Mr. America, which was disappointing, especially considering that I had won the Mr. Western Hemisphere just 6 weeks before. But shortly after that, I rebounded and won Mr. South. My next contest was the AAU Mr. USA in August 1970 in New Orleans. I thought I had a good chance of winning, or at least placing high.

As I approached the exhibition hall, where the competition was held, up walked Casey Viator. I knew him well enough; he lived near Boyer Coe in Louisiana, and we'd competed against each other several times. He placed fourth in the 1969 Mr. Texas and second in the 1970 Mr. Western Hemisphere. But 6 weeks later, he finished third at the Mr. America. (Chris Dickerson won.)

My 4 years of national-level bodybuilding competitions made me believe that Viator's third-place finish was a fluke. After all, he was just 18, and it was rare for someone to finish in the top five at a national contest in his first try. The last four Mr. America winners—Dickerson, Coe, Jim Haislop, and Dennis Tinerino—had all worked their way up to the top through multiple tries.

But when I saw Viator on that sweltering August day in New Orleans, he looked huge. "What in the world have you been doing?" I questioned.

"Ask him," he said, pointing to a nondescript, balding man with a mustache. "Ask Arthur Jones."

But before I could introduce myself to Jones, much less ask detailed questions about his training methods, he gave me my first order. "Come over here and give us a hand," Jones said to me and the other bodybuilders standing around. It wasn't a request.

All of us followed Jones and Viator around to the back of the building, where a small trailer was parked next to a loading dock. Inside the trailer were several welded metal frames painted blue, along with some cables, black upholstered benches, and hundreds of pounds of barbell plates.

Jones began barking orders: "Separate those pieces, grab these bolts and a wrench, stack that part on top of this one, turn the whole thing around, and screw the seat in place."

In less than 5 minutes, we had it together. "Now put 150 pounds of plates on the back side," Jones said.

Over that 5-minute period, my mind ran through everything I knew about Jones. I was aware of his articles in *IronMan.* I'd seen his huge machine at the Mr. America. What I didn't know was that Jones had talked Viator into relocating to Florida and had been training him for most of the summer. But what I did know was that there was something very different about Viator. As we worked up a

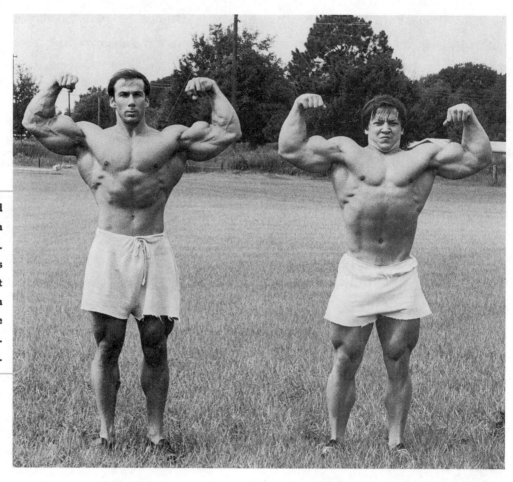

Boyer Coe and Casey Viator in October 1970. Arthur Jones was just starting to train Viator for the 1971 Mr. America.

sweat under the 90-degree midday sun, with the New Orleans humidity right at the dew point, I kept noticing the vascularity of Viator's arms, which looked several inches larger than mine.

Jones Clues Me In

"Okay, Ell Darden, belt yourself into the seat, and I'll teach you something about exercise," Jones said.

"Teach *me* something about exercise?" I thought. I'd almost completed my course work for a Ph.D. in exercise science. It seemed as if it should've been the other way around. Still, I went along, belting myself into the seat of his pullover

machine and starting the movement. The barbell pullover was sort of a specialty of mine, so the exercise felt somewhat redundant to me.

"How does this exercise differ from the barbell pullover?" I asked, as I knocked out 3 or 4 repetitions.

Before I knew it, Jones was lecturing me on why his machine provided rotary resistance and a barbell didn't. As a result, none of the other guys got a chance to try the machine. Viator, standing in the background, laughed at me. He knew how big a can of worms I was opening.

When I unbelted myself from the machine, Jones asked about my university studies, and I told him about being close to finishing a Ph.D. at Florida State. Then he said something that eventually changed my life.

"You think you're pretty smart, don't you, Ell Darden?" (For some reason, Jones wouldn't call me Ellington, or Ell, or Darden; it was always Ell Darden.) And before I could answer, or even shrug, he went off: "If you can unlearn everything you've learned about exercise—and you can do this un-learning before you reach age 40—you'll be headed in the right direction. Then, after you reach 40, you just may be in the position where you can learn something of real value. And, if you do, you'll in-deed be smart."

At the time, I had no idea how critical those words would turn out to be. But over the next dozen years, what he said became plainer and plainer in my personal quest for knowledge. I can truly say that I have a far greater understanding of my chosen field now than I did then. And, true to Jones's prophecy, I achieved this by first unlearning just about everything I thought I had understood about exercise.

Jones invited me to visit him in Lake Helen, which was about 270 miles south of the campus in Tallahassee. "You can see for yourself the way Casey's been exercising," he said. "The key, however, is a very high intensity of effort and the avoidance of overtraining."

I wasn't sure what he meant. But I sure wasn't going to ask and risk getting another lecture. I needed to retreat and get some rest and ready my-self for the contest.

That night, Casey Viator looked amazing and won the 1970 Mr. USA. Clearly, his success at the

Mr. America back in June had been no fluke. When I failed to place in the top 10, I decided to take Arthur Jones up on his offer.

Queasy at the Quonset Hut

I called Jones a week later and told him I wanted to visit. The next day, I drove to Lake Helen, where I met with him for 6 consecutive hours. The high-light was a workout in a Quonset hut at DeLand High School, where Jones kept his machines. The original Blue Monster had now been redesigned into four separate machines, which were much more practical and functional.

Jones put me through a lat cycle and an arm cycle. The entire workout consisted of seven move-ments, one set of each, with limited rest between the exercises.

On each exercise, when I thought I was finished, Jones would say, "Don't stop; get another repeti-tion." I ended up getting 3 more repetitions on most of them, plus a final assisted rep with Jones's help. For the first time, I was experiencing *outright hard work*. After about 10 minutes, I was cooked. Jones wanted to put me on a final leg cycle, but there was no way I could have finished it.

I lay flat on my stomach on a cool concrete floor for 3 minutes, until I felt better. Jones helped me stand up, and we both noted that my arms were thoroughly pumped. Afterward, I was sore through-out my lats, biceps, and triceps for 3 days.

Back in Tallahassee, I reread all of Jones's arti-cles in *IronMan*. And when he sent me his self-published manual, called *Nautilus Training Principles, Bulletin No. 1,* I read that, too—all 44 chapters and 60,000 words. Still, I wasn't ready to go all the way over to the high-intensity side. I experimented with it on a few exercises but nothing more.

A Workout to Write About

In May 1971, I decided to skip the Mr. America competition, which was to be held the following month in York, Pennsylvania. Casey Viator was getting a huge amount of publicity, including photographs, from Jones's articles in *IronMan*. I figured he would be almost impossible to beat.

So I accepted Jones's invitation to watch Viator's last workout before they left for the contest. I wasn't the only spectator. Elliott Plese, Ph.D., of Colorado State University was there. So was Kim Wood, a former football player and strength athlete from the University of Wisconsin, who'd been hired by Jones to help with the training at the Quonset hut. Larry Gilmore was there to help keep Viator focused during his workout. On the night of June 10, 1971, two days before the Mr. America, we watched Viator do the following routine:

1. Leg press on Universal machine, 750 pounds, for 20 repetitions, immediately followed by

2. Leg extension on Universal machine, 225 pounds for 20 repetitions, immediately followed by

3. Full squat with barbell, 502 pounds for 13 repetitions. He rested for 2 minutes and drank water.

4. Leg curl on Universal machine, 175 pounds for 12 repetitions, immediately followed by

5. One-legged calf raise with a 40-pound dumbbell held in one hand, first one leg and then the other, 15 repetitions for each leg, immediately followed by

6. Pullover on Nautilus machine, 290 pounds for 11 repetitions, immediately followed by

7. Behind-the-neck lat-isolation exercise on Nautilus machine, 200 pounds for 10 repetitions, immediately followed by

8. Rowing on Nautilus machine, 200 pounds for 10 repetitions, immediately followed by

9. Behind-the-neck lat pulldown on Nautilus machine, 210 pounds for 10 repetitions. He rested for 2 minutes and drank water.

10. Straight-armed lateral raise with dumbbells, 40 pounds in each hand for 9 repetitions, immediately followed by

11. Behind-the-neck shoulder press with barbell, 185 pounds for 10 repetitions. He rested for 2 minutes and drank water.

12. Biceps curl on Nautilus plate-loading machine, 110 pounds for 8 repetitions, immediately followed by

13. Chinup, using his own body weight for 12 repetitions. He rested for 2 minutes and drank water.

14. Triceps extension on Nautilus plate-loading machine, 125 pounds for 9 repetitions, immediately followed by

15. Parallel dip, using his own body weight for 22 repetitions.

Jones pushed Viator through each exercise, and every set was carried to the point of momentary muscular failure. The leg cycle, exercises 1 through 5, took 10 minutes. The upper-body routine, exercises 6 through 15, including rest periods, took 17 minutes and 40 seconds. The entire workout, from start to finish, required exactly 27 minutes and 40 seconds.

According to Jones, who'd been training Viator for 10 months, this was his best workout yet. That wasn't much of a surprise, because it was the most amazing workout I'd ever witnessed. But then Jones said something truly startling: Over the last 4 weeks, Viator had trained only six times. That's right, only six times in 28 days.

I couldn't decide which was more impressive: the weight Viator handled on these exercises (par-ticularly the leg press and squat) or the cardiorespi-ratory condition that he must have had in order to go from one exercise to the next without rest.

Jones asked Viator to take off his T-shirt, which was dripping with sweat. Viator contracted his right biceps, then his left, then turned around and hit a back double-biceps pose. I'd never seen such mus-cular density.

As I drove back to Tallahassee, I was certain that Casey Viator would win the 1971 Mr. America. What I didn't know was the extraordinary way he would accomplish this goal.

Chapter 3

THE YOUNGEST-EVER MR. AMERICA

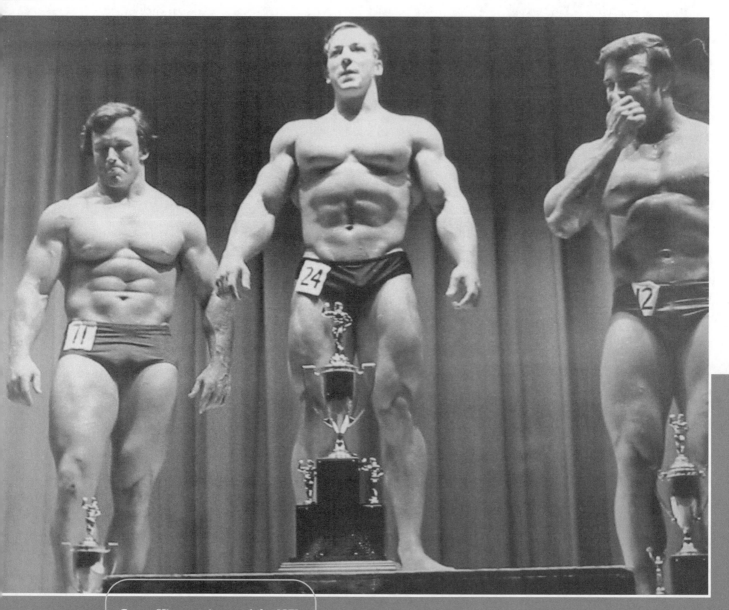

Casey Viator, winner of the 1971 AAU Mr. America, is flanked by (left to right) Bill St. John (third) and Pete Grymkowski (second).

"YOU HAVEN'T HEARD yet who won?" Jones said, when I finally got him on the phone after several days of trying. It was June 17, 1971, and in those pre-Internet days, word didn't travel as fast. "Thirty-three men entered. Casey was the 24th man to pose. It was over after that—Casey was an easy winner."

"Who was second?"

"Pete Grymkowski, a guy with huge deltoids," Jones said. "He was the only competitor who weighed more than Casey, but he didn't have anything close to Casey's shape and definition."

Jones told me Casey Viator weighed 218 pounds at just under 5 feet 8 inches. Grymkowski, who was 5 feet 10½ inches, claimed a body weight of 232 pounds, but Jones guessed that he really weighed 225.

When I got my hands on the official contest report that was later published, I saw Viator had scored 377 points from the eight judges. Grymkowski was next with 350 points, followed by Bill St. John, Ed Corney, and Carl Smith. In 10th place was Mike Mentzer, who later became one of the most forceful proponents for high-intensity training. (I'll tell some of his story in chapter 9.)

Interestingly, in national bodybuilding competitions at that time, there were six different subdivisions aside from the Mr. America title. There was a contest for most muscular, which was judged on having the best combination of size, vascularity, and leanness. Then there were separate contests for best arms, best chest, best abdominals, best back, and best legs. Maybe a guy couldn't compete successfully in the overall title of Mr. America, but with a pair of magnificent arms or great legs, for example, he could still win or place in one of these subdivi-

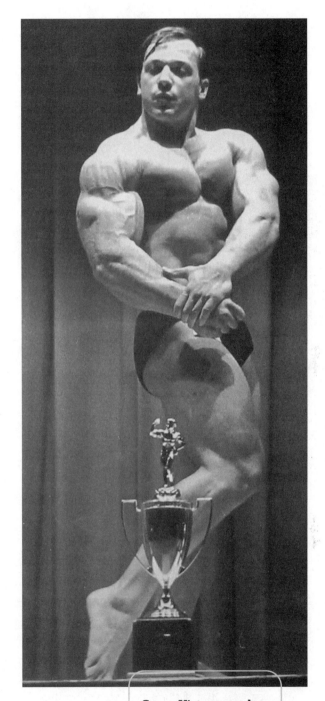

Casey Viator was also winner of the 1971 Mr. America subdivisions Most Muscular, Best Arms, Best Chest, Best Back, and Best Legs.

Clearing the Air of Steroids

Big, cut, vascular, and only 19 years old. Those words accurately described Casey Viator as he won the 1971 Mr. America. Some wanted to know what kind of program he used, but many had a different question: "What drug cycles is Casey on?"

I'll make this as clear as possible: Arthur Jones was, and still is, against bodybuilding steroids. In one of his early training manuals, *Nautilus Training Principles, Bulletin No. 2*, he wrote: "If you are using drugs—of any kind—don't bother to come to DeLand, Florida, hoping to train; and please don't be foolish enough to think you can fool me on the subject—even though you might, briefly."

Jones then vowed to do "that which is necessary" to make sure that steroids don't infiltrate the high-intensity training gym in DeLand. A few bodybuilders, in fact, learned the hard way that Jones meant what he said.

Concerning Viator, Jones told me that when he relocated to Florida in the summer of 1970, Viator gave his word that he wouldn't take steroids. When asked about being on drugs leading up to his 1971 Mr. America victory, Viator flatly denied using them, and Jones always respected his denial. I think Jones would have severed his relationship with Viator if he'd even suspected his famous pupil was on steroids.

I don't have any laboratory analyses to prove Viator was or wasn't taking steroids in 1970 and 1971. But I trust Jones and Viator. I was around both of them for many years, and I firmly believe Viator grew bigger, stronger, and more vascular because of his high-intensity training and his unusual genetic potential—and not from drugs.

Jones was consistent with his view of steroid use in bodybuilding: He thought that the benefits were overrated while the side effects were underrated. But he did make one famous exception. When he trained Sergio Oliva for 6 weeks in 1971, Oliva was on steroids and Jones knew it. Here's what he wrote about that: "If Sergio went off the drugs, he would undoubtedly lose muscular size for at least 6 months, until such time that his body was able to return to a normal chemical balance.

"Sergio is an exceptional case. I don't approve of his use of such drugs, but I will at least permit it under the circumstances. However, there will be no other such exceptions. So if you have been using these drugs, I would advise you to cease their use at least 6 months before even seriously considering coming to DeLand to train."

Years later, Jones asked Boyer Coe and Mike and Ray Mentzer to promise him that they wouldn't take steroids during their employment with Nautilus. Jones said that each gave him his word.

sions. Many bodybuilders of that day took great pride in saying they had been finalists in the Best Arms, Best Abs, or Best Chest division of the Mr. America.

Viator won five of the six subdivisions in 1971, and according to just about every witness I've spoken to, no one really came close to him in those five. His only loss was Best Abdominals, and even in that subdivision he was one of the finalists. No one in the history of the Mr. America had won that many awards.

And Viator was only 19, competing against men who, on average, were 9½ years older.

The Challenge

I decided to spend August 1971 in DeLand, training under Jones's supervision. Jones was now manufacturing at least six exercise machines, which he called Nautilus. I slept in a spare bedroom.

Before I went to DeLand, I had applied some of Jones's concepts to my own workouts by doing the following:

- Training my entire body during each workout

- Selecting only 12 basic exercises to perform

- Performing each exercise in a high-intensity manner, or until no more repetitions were possible

- Limiting each exercise to two sets

- Repeating the workout three times per week

When I told Jones what I was doing, he suggested I reduce my workouts even further. "Do two sets of 10 exercises, and you'll get even better results."

After 2 weeks, with special attention paid to my form, I realized that I needed to cut the routine even more—which is exactly what Jones hoped would happen. I settled on a routine of two sets of eight exercises, performed three times per week. My body responded, and 7 months later, on April 23, 1972, I won the last national contest that I entered: Collegiate Mr. America.

I weighed 195 pounds at 5 feet 11 inches, and I figured I'd gone as far as my muscular potential would allow.

Positive Thoughts about the Negative

During a visit with Jones in July 1972, I shared an article I'd written for a fitness magazine on using mud as a source of resistance. Mud resistance seemed ideal for working the small muscles of the hands and feet. Jones then made a point that I'd never considered before. "The problem with mud resistance is that it provides no negative work. And without negative work, an exercise is of limited value."

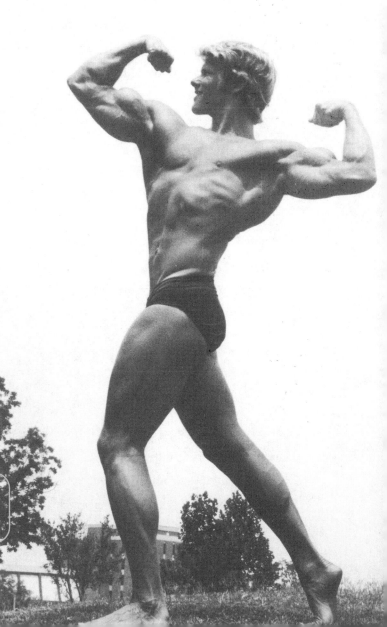

This photo was taken several days after I won the 1972 Collegiate Mr. America.

Jones was correct. Mud exercise was similar to water exercise. When you stand submerged to your shoulders in water (or mud) and do an open-handed biceps curl, you feel it in your biceps muscle. But once in the contracted position, there's little negative resistance on the lowering. In fact, if you really force your arm to extend, you're doing so with your triceps. So water or mud exercise supplies positive-only work.

A month later, something amazing happened. I was in Munich, Germany, at a scientific conference preceding the 1972 Olympics. In one of the sessions, Dr. Paavo Komi, a Finnish physiologist, described how he had trained a small group of Scandinavian weight lifters by having them lower—not lift—heavier-than-normal barbells from overhead to the floor. His study then compared the effects of positive and negative work on the electrical activity of human muscle. He was convinced that his negative training of the Scandinavian weight lifters just might provide them with an edge in their approaching Olympic competition. Several days later, one of Dr. Komi's athletes won a gold medal and two won bronzes.

I told Dr. Komi I was interested in his ongoing research and wanted to keep in touch with him. I also mentioned that I would soon be working with Arthur Jones of Nautilus Sports/Medical Industries. Dr. Komi told me he'd experimented with using various hydraulic machines to help with the lifting of extremely heavy barbells for his athletes, but the machines had been difficult to use.

When I returned from Europe, I called Jones and told him about Dr. Komi and his research with negative work. "Bring those reports down to me imme-diately," Jones said. (We didn't have fax machines in those days.) "I have some new developments that I want to show you."

Doing "Negatives"

The first thing Jones did when I arrived in Lake Helen was drive me to the high school for a workout—his workout. Jones was back in training, but this time he was doing it in a negative-only style, which involved some brand-new concepts. Another assistant and I helped Jones perform one set of 10 repetitions of the following exercises:

• Nautilus pullover, negative only

• Nautilus torso-arm pulldown to chest, negative only

• Barbell bench press, negative only

• Barbell curl, normal positive and negative

• Nautilus triceps extension, negative only

• Nautilus biceps curl, negative only

• Parallel dip, negative only

• Barbell wrist curl, negative only

Eight exercises, and seven of them were done negative only, with weights that were about 50 percent heavier than he could normally lift for 10 repetitions. We did all the lifting—the positive work—for him. Then we transferred the resistance to his arms, and he did the lowering—the negative work. He took 8 to 10 seconds to lower the weight on each repetition. On the parallel dip, he placed a sturdy chair in front of the dip bars so that he could step into the top position before lowering himself.

According to Jones, this was his sixth workout in the past 11 days, and his arms had already grown by $\frac{7}{8}$ inch. At the end of 14 days, he expected his arms to have increased by a full inch as a result of those six very brief workouts. (That's exactly what happened.)

After a short trip to the Tastee-Freez for a milkshake, Jones drove me to his new prototype shop in Lake Helen for a look at some new machines. On the way, I went over the reports that Dr. Komi had given to the Olympic Congress attendees. Jones was disappointed that Dr. Komi was so tentative in his conclusions. "There's no doubt in my mind that for the purpose of building muscular size and strength, negative work is far more important than positive work. I don't yet know exactly why negative work is so effective. But I'm going to find out soon."

Just then, we pulled up to the Nautilus prototype shop in Lake Helen. Inside were at least five prototypes for machines that Jones was calling Omni. I couldn't help being amazed. He'd come a long way from the Blue Monster in just 2 years.

There were separate machines for the shoulders, chest, biceps, and triceps, and one for multiple applications, including chinning and dipping. Each piece of equipment had a foot pedal incorporated into the machine, which provided the user with a way to lift a heavier-than-normal resistance with his legs so that he could lower it with his torso or arms.

Jones launched into a lecture. "As you probably have realized by now, Ell Darden, during a negative-only routine, it's difficult to find spotters to do the lifting for you consistently. You just assisted me through an upper-body workout. I'm nowhere as strong as Casey or some of our other athletes. And with heavy weights, and two or more guys trying to lift and transfer the load smoothly to the trainee, there's the danger of getting injured if there's a slip or miscommunication. These new Omni machines will allow the trainee to be in control.

"When they're completed, we're going to do some major research in university settings to demonstrate clearly the value of negative work."

Nine months later, at the 1973 Mr. America contest, I learned the results of one of those studies.

The Colorado Experiment

In early January 1973, Casey Viator weighed $200\frac{1}{2}$ pounds and was working nights at a wire-extruding plant in DeLand. A serious accident at the plant caused him to lose most of the little finger of his right hand. Several days later, he almost died from an allergic reaction to an anti-tetanus injection. He was nauseated and depressed for the next $3\frac{1}{2}$ months and didn't train. He had little appetite. His muscles atrophied, and he lost more than 33 pounds, with $18\frac{3}{4}$ of the pounds being attributed to the nearly fatal injection.

Jones recognized that Viator needed to get back into training—the sooner, the better. He put on hold a plan to exercise dozens of subjects in a major strength-training project and instead decided to use Viator as a case study.

He sent his latest machines to Colorado State University in Fort Collins, had them assembled in the exercise physiology laboratory, and then flew there with Viator to start training on May 1, 1973, with the study to conclude on May 29. The training would be monitored by Elliott Plese, Ph.D.

Jones, of course, believed that muscular growth was related to the intensity of exercise. If the intensity was high enough, then a large amount of training was neither necessary nor desirable. Jones's plan was to train Viator hard and briefly: one set to failure of 12 or fewer exercises, repeated progressively every other day, for 4 weeks.

Viator's body weight increased from 166.87 pounds to 212.15 pounds, for an overall gain of 45.28 pounds. Body-composition analysis (using the then-state-of-the-art potassium-40, whole-body counter), revealed that Viator had actually built significantly more muscle than his gain in body weight indicated. Over the 28-day period, he had lost 17.93 pounds of fat; his percentage of body fat went from 13.8 to 2.47. That meant he had actually built 63.21 pounds of muscle . . . in just 28 days.

You've probably heard the saying that if something seems too good to be true, it probably is. Jones realized this as well as anybody. No one would believe that a human could gain 2.25 pounds of muscle a day for 28 days. That's why Jones was always careful to point out that, prior to the study, Viator had been in a disabling accident and his

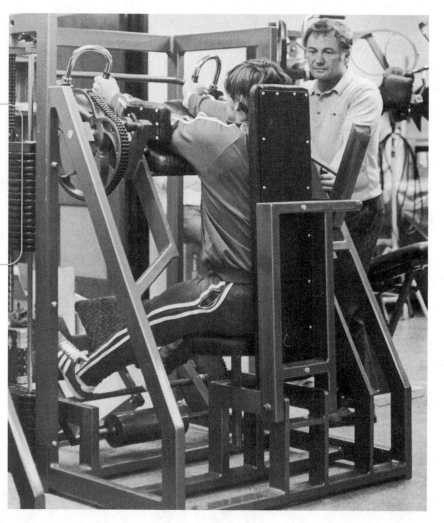

Dr. Elliott Plese of Colorado State University observes as Casey Viator performs a set on the Nautilus Omni triceps machine. A foot-pedal attachment allowed Viator to do the positive work with his legs.

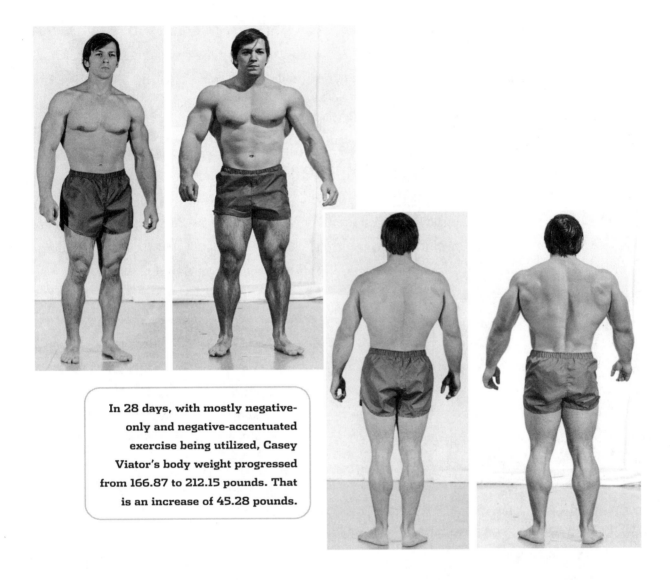

In 28 days, with mostly negative-only and negative-accentuated exercise being utilized, Casey Viator's body weight progressed from 166.87 to 212.15 pounds. That is an increase of 45.28 pounds.

muscles had atrophied. Thus, during the study, he was *rebuilding* previously existing levels of muscular size.

Jones had a full report, with pictures, of the Colorado experiment in the next issue of *IronMan*. He was sure to point out that more than half of the total sets that Casey Viator performed were done in either a negative-only fashion, where the resistance was lowered only, or a negative-accentuated manner, where the resistance was raised with both limbs and then lowered with only one limb.

Until Jones became involved with negative work in 1972, no one paid much attention to the lowering phase of an exercise. During the entire 1960s, I had never heard a trainee talk about "doing negatives." Now, thanks to Arthur Jones, "doing negatives" is a normal part of a bodybuilder's training lexicon.

Fit to Print

Peary Rader, editor and publisher of *IronMan*, had his headquarters in Alliance, Nebraska, which is 225 miles northeast of Fort Collins. Jones flew up there one morning and toured Rader's facilities. Besides printing *IronMan,* Rader also printed a number of other magazines throughout the Midwest and owned the distributorship for the European printing equipment that he used in his shop. Talking to Rader and seeing his operation gave Jones the idea to jump into the printing business and do all of Nautilus's brochures, catalogs, and advertising—even a magazine, eventually—in-house. Rader said he'd get Jones a good deal on all the necessary equipment and even volunteered to train two of Jones's people for 6 weeks.

I was one of those people. I had just a month to go in my yearlong postdoctoral study at Florida State's nutrition department, so I accepted Jones's offer.

I left for Nebraska in mid-July 1973 with Inge Toppenwien Cook, a longtime employee of Jones's. It was a fascinating 6 weeks. Not only did I learn how to operate multiple printing presses, but I also got to spend a lot of time with Rader, who'd been involved in bodybuilding and strength training for more than 50 years.

He also had what might've been the best library of bodybuilding publications in the world at that time, with collections of muscle magazines going back to the early 1900s. I took a stack of books and magazines back to the local hotel with me each night.

When Inge and I returned to Lake Helen in September, the Nautilus headquarters was bustling. Multiple buildings were under construction, including one that would house a training room. Jones had already hired a printer and graphic artist, in anticipation of the presses and auxiliary equipment arriving the following week. We were about to go into the publishing business.

We desperately needed materials concerning guidelines, routines, adaptations, and applications. More than 20 different Nautilus machines were now being manufactured, sold, and shipped throughout the United States. And bodybuilders, football players, coaches, and medical doctors were showing up in Lake Helen on a weekly basis to learn more about high-intensity training.

Jones had made a simple promise: "I'll personally meet with everyone, and if need be, I'll personally train anyone who's man enough to do what I say." In the December 1971 issue of *IronMan,* under the headline "Now—Train Under the Personal Direction of Arthur Jones," he made this boast: "Within the last year, our trainees have won 34 first-place trophies. We must be doing something right."

He had a point, but Nautilus was now too big for Jones to continue doing it as a one-man show. Someone needed to step up, and, as I'll explain in the next chapter, one of those people turned out to be me.

Chapter 4

HIT HAPPENS!

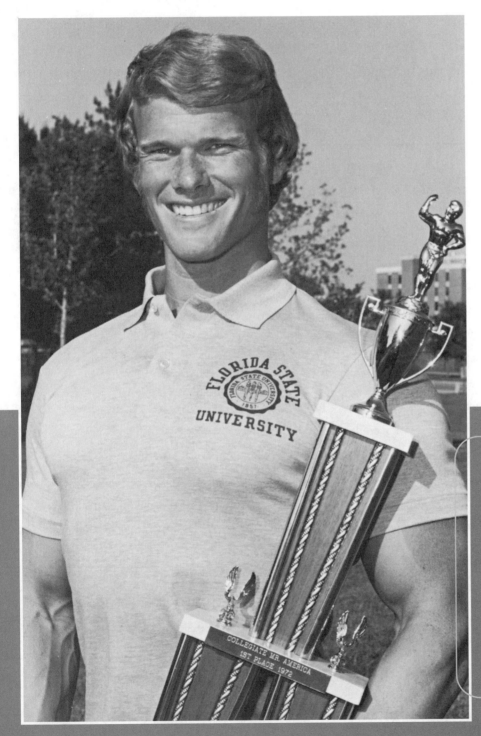

While studying exercise science and nutrition in graduate school at Florida State University, I won the 1972 Collegiate Mr. America title; and in my course work, I excelled at being concise and organized. These traits prepared me to blend well with Arthur Jones.

IN LATE NOVEMBER 1975, I had officially been working for Arthur Jones for more than 2 years. But a lot had happened since I met him in 1970. Along with the milestones I've already described—Casey Viator winning the 1971 Mr. America, me winning the 1972 Collegiate Mr. America—the Miami Dolphins went undefeated and won the Super Bowl in 1973, after buying into high-intensity training. They successfully defended their title in 1974.

Other sports teams soon bought full sets of Nautilus machines: the Cincinnati Bengals, Houston Oilers, Boston Celtics, New York Yankees, Cincinnati Reds. Three top college programs—the University of Alabama, the University of Notre Dame, and the University of Texas—did so as well.

But something was still missing. Too many people were confused about what exactly we were promoting. And Jones, for all his brilliance, was often adding to the confusion with his discursive anecdotes, gross generalizations, and sometimes-complex transitions from one topic to the next.

In graduate school, I'd learned the value of concise language. If you couldn't make a point quickly and move on, you got marked down.

Jones's instinct to be all over the place, and my newly acquired ability to organize my thoughts and present them concisely, would soon merge in a completely unexpected way.

Fighting Words

Duke University had just purchased a line of Nautilus machines for their sports complex, and Jones decided he would personally explain to the faculty and interested students the philosophy behind the equipment. So Duke organized a one-day seminar. I traveled to North Carolina with a small group that included Jones, Viator, Dick Butkus, and a handful of others.

Jones hadn't counted on the structure and formality of the seminar. An interested history professor had divided the seminar into six 1-hour time blocks, with a break for lunch in the middle. The topics to be covered during those time blocks were the following: the history of exercise, high-intensity philosophy, training equipment, training principles, routines, and the future of exercise.

Each 1-hour time block had a planned format: 30 minutes of lecture, a 5-minute summary, a 10-minute question-and-answer session, a 5-minute critique from a graduate student, and then a 10-minute break. And to make it even more awkward, the professor had assumed that all of us traveling with Jones would participate, with each of us taking charge of a 1-hour time block.

No setup could have been less suited to Arthur Jones. He dislikes formality, has trouble remembering names, seldom shakes hands, never wears a tie, dismisses small talk, and, above all else, hates being told that he has to follow someone else's itinerary.

Jones planned to do all the lectures himself and maybe, after a couple of hours, have Viator take his shirt off and hit front and back double-biceps poses. Or maybe Dick Butkus, because he was a famous All-Pro football player, would be asked to stand up and take a bow. That was it. The rest was to be the Arthur Jones show.

The professor introduced Jones, and as soon as Jones started speaking, we were in trouble with this audience. He started with a story about the differ-

What Happened to the Mr. America Contest?

From 1940 to 1973, the most prestigious bodybuilding contest in the world was the AAU Mr. America. Even if you're just a casual fan of bodybuilding, you'll recognize the names of many of the winners: John Grimek (1940), Clancy Ross (1945), Steve Reeves (1947), George Eiferman (1948), Bill Pearl (1953), Red Lerille (1960), Boyer Coe (1969), Chris Dickerson (1970), and, of course, Casey Viator (1971). There were other contests: The National Amateur Bodybuilders Association (NABBA) had its annual Mr. Universe in London, and the International Federation of Bodybuilding (IFBB—Joe and Ben Weider's organization) had its Mr. America and Mr. Universe. But the AAU still had the most-coveted competitions.

That began to change in the mid-1970s. Bob Hoffman, founder of York Barbell and publisher of *Strength and Health* magazine, had been a prominent promoter of the AAU Mr. America. But he was in declining health, while Joe Weider was gaining influence. Weider's bodybuilding magazines, now featuring rising star Arnold Schwarzenegger, were more popular than ever. But perhaps more important in the decline of the Mr. America was the rise of another contest.

Weider created the Mr. Olympia in 1965 as a professional bodybuilding show, reserved only for the present and past champions. The first contest included Mr. America (Dave Draper) and Mr. Universe (Earl Maynard), and was won by Larry Scott, who had previously won those two titles and Mr. World for good measure. The prize money was small at first—barely $1,000—and the contest was not always a "contest" in the strictest sense. Sergio Oliva won it unopposed in 1968, as did Schwarzenegger in 1971, when all the top competitors went to London for the NABBA Mr. Universe. But the prize money gradually increased (today it's over $100,000), and it's now acknowledged as the most important title in professional bodybuilding. Running a close second to the Mr. Olympia is the Arnold Classic, a professional contest that Schwarzenegger started in 1989 and that has the endorsement of the IFBB.

So what became of the Mr. America? Its prestige gradually fell, especially after the formation of the National Physique Committee (NPC) in 1982. Today, the NPC sanctions state, regional, and national contests, and NPC national winners are eligible to receive IFBB "pro cards," which means they can compete for the big titles—and big money.

With the rise of the NPC, and its affiliation with the Weiders' IFBB, the AAU Mr. America was discontinued in 1999. A lot of bodybuilding history went down with the Mr. America. State titles such as Mr. Florida, Mr. Texas, and Mr. California no longer exist. And hundreds of local contests—Mr. Pittsburgh, Mr. New Orleans, Mr. Atlanta—also went by the wayside.

---

ence between being ignorant and being stupid:

"We're all ignorant because there are many concepts that we are not familiar with. If I'm in the possession of some valuable information that you don't have, then I'm at fault if I don't make it available to you. But once I explain the material in a clear, logical manner, then the new pathway should be self-evident to an elementary school student or even a chimpanzee.

"On the other hand, if, after you've heard the facts and had time to reflect, you've chosen to ignore or reject them, that's your fault.

"Now, you are no longer ignorant. You're stupid. And stupidity goes clear to the bone!"

Jones said he could deal with ignorance, but he had no patience for stupidity. "Stupidity just might get you a personal escort—by me—to the back alley for a good ass-kicking."

No one in the Duke University audience had heard such an abrupt opening to a seminar. The attendees didn't know whether to laugh or walk out.

I'd like to say that Jones lightened up after the opening, but he didn't. His lecture got more serious. He spewed facts and figures. He intimidated with words and actions. He picked on the people in the front rows. He embarrassed those in the back rows for being afraid to sit down front. He insulted the ones in the middle for being . . . in the middle.

This went on for 3 hours. There were no 10-minute question-and-answer periods. There were no refreshment breaks. There was no escape from Jones's unrelenting drive to get his point across.

Finally, the history professor stood up and sheepishly suggested that we break for lunch. After lunch, we'd begin with the critiques. A tall, thin man with long hair spoke up. He was supposed to critique the second topic, high-intensity philosophy. He couldn't return after lunch and asked if he could share his remarks now.

"Yes," Jones said. "I'm all ears."

The young man, a Ph.D. candidate in physics, had a long list of issues with Jones's theories. He rambled on for several minutes before Jones cut him off. He told the young man that he liked to do only two things: lecture and fistfight. Did the man want to do the latter, either before or after lunch?

The challenge drew catcalls from the audience, while the grad student (wisely) disappeared.

Saved by the Ell

Ralph Nader, the consumer advocate, was speaking nearby. Our group mingled with theirs during the lunch break, and many who had started the day listening to Nader decided to finish it watching the combustible Jones. In addition, many of those who'd witnessed Jones in action in the morning told friends to come see the second-half fireworks.

At the end of the lunch break—which stretched to 2 hours—we had a much bigger audience than the original group, and one that was now primed for action.

Jones picked up where he'd left off. He had heard that his critic from the morning had been a protester of the Vietnam War and had hidden out in Canada for several years to avoid being drafted. Jones graphically described what he would've done to the young man, after he'd thoroughly whipped his ass in the alley.

The thought of ripping the man to pieces seemed to mellow Jones a bit, and he offered to take questions from the audience. After 15 uneventful minutes of this, he brought Viator on stage, telling him to take off his shirt and flex his arms. The audience enjoyed that part and asked a few more questions, mostly about bodybuilding.

But Jones then veered off again. He talked about his experiences in Africa for almost an hour, then went off on Ralph Nader for a while, then returned to his Congo River adventures and his take on the Rhodesian range wars.

The audience was weary, and the poor professor who'd arranged all this was afraid to allow Jones to continue much longer. He waited for the first pause in Jones's monologue and then called for a 15-minute break. Then he tapped me on the shoulder and motioned me over.

"Ellington, can you please get up in front of

this audience and summarize high-intensity exercise?" The professor asked if, at the very least, I could offer some guidelines for using the Nautilus equipment.

I told him I could.

"Good. I want you to start in 10 minutes. Get up there, introduce yourself, and start summarizing." He promised to distract Jones until I had a good head of steam. He made it clear that I was the last hope for salvaging an otherwise disastrous seminar.

Luckily for me, in the third through sixth grades, my parents had given me the choice of taking piano lessons or taking "expression." Expression was learning how to stand and give a speech. At that time in my life, I had no interest in making speeches. But I had less interest in learning to play the piano. That, I figured, was for sissies. So I took expression for 3 long years, after which I knew how to stand up straight, look my audience in the eyes, and project my voice in an interesting manner.

Luckily for me, from the research and writing I had done at Florida State, I knew how to organize subject matter into parallel headings and subheadings.

Luckily for me, for the past 3 years, I had read everything that was available concerning high-intensity exercise and Nautilus guidelines.

No one, especially Arthur Jones, knew that I was prepared to speak on high-intensity training. But I was ready.

The professor headed toward Jones and his entourage, and I retreated to the restroom. We both had a lot to think about and very little time.

Five minutes later, as the crowd was shuffling back to their seats, I stepped up to the lectern.

Halfway through my brief introduction, I saw the history professor, Jones, and Viator appear at the top of the stairs. We were in one of those auditoriums where the seats rise in a semicircle around a lectern and blackboard. I saw Jones frown as he started down the stairs, with the professor desperately trying to hold his attention.

I turned my back to the audience, picked up a piece of chalk, and wrote in big block letters on the blackboard:

HIGH-INTENSITY TRAINING

Underneath this heading, I wrote:

INTENSITY

PROGRESSION

FORM

DURATION

FREQUENCY

ORDER

When I turned around, I saw that Jones, Viator, and the professor had taken seats in the middle of the audience, directly in front of me. I could read the look on Jones's face: "Screw up, and I'll kick your butt all the way back to Florida." The professor looked as if he hoped for a miracle but didn't expect one. Viator, on the other hand, wore a big smile. Even though we were past our posedown days, there was still some competitiveness between us. The expression on his face told me that he couldn't wait to see me squirm.

But I didn't. To tell you the truth, I don't think I've ever given a better talk, and I've spoken in front of groups hundreds of times since that day.

I discussed intensity for 3 minutes. I made a smooth transition to the concept of progression.

The Wry Wit of Arthur Jones

Unless you've heard Arthur Jones speak to a large group of bodybuilders and strength professionals—it's difficult to appreciate his humor, jest, and ability to entertain a crowd. Below, collected over 25 years, are some of his most amusing quips.

● If you *like* an exercise, chances are you're doing it wrong.

● A properly performed set of leg extensions immediately followed by a properly performed set of leg presses should leave you feeling like you just climbed a tall building with your car tied to your back.

● We learn, when we learn, only from experience, and then we only learn from our mistakes. Our successes only serve to reinforce our superstitions.

● Never be so arrogant that you fail to give people the benefit of being as stupid as they actually are.

● Thinking is a terrible disadvantage with which most people are not burdened. Being able to think merely makes you aware of the outrages around you.

● How would you feel if you lived on an island populated, apart from yourself, exclusively by retarded, malicious chimpanzees? Well, that's how I feel. Don't laugh, because you're one of those retarded, malicious chimpanzees.

● Voting for politicians who tell you what you want to hear has all but destroyed civilization, giving in to outrage in the hope of avoiding trouble has all but destroyed freedom, and looking for the *easy* road to success in bodybuilding has all but destroyed the actually great potential value of weight training.

● If racehorses were trained as much as most bodybuilders train, you could safely bet your money on an out-of-condition turtle.

● Split routines make about as much sense as sleeping with one eye open. Best results will almost always occur from exercising both your upper body and your lower body in the same workout.

● There must surely be a few bodybuilders who are not idiots. But if so, they are well camouflaged in some undiscovered cave.

● How old am I? Old enough to know it's impossible to change the thinking of fools, but young and foolish enough to keep on trying.

Jones and the professor seemed to relax. Viator was smiling and shaking his head at the same time, like he couldn't believe that I was actually pulling it off.

But I was.

At one point, Jones even raised his hand and asked me a question about protein requirements for athletes. That opened the door for more questions about nutrition and its role in strength training.

I talked for approximately 40 minutes, with enthusiastic audience participation in the last half.

It seems strange to say now, but my outline represented the first time that Jones's high-intensity concepts had been condensed, separated, and concisely stated. I even used the acronym "HIT" several times, which was another first. HIT was born that day.

We were in the air, heading back to Florida, less than an hour after the professor closed the seminar. In case you're wondering, I never heard anything from the professor after that. I imagine he vowed to himself that he'd never have anything to do with another strength-training seminar.

Pearl Jam

Four years later, Jones finally told me what he thought about my performance at Duke. We were in a van, heading to a New York airport, reminiscing about a party in which I'd been hit in the face by a cream pie. Jones said he was impressed by the fact that I controlled my reaction and didn't try to retaliate. "You know, Ell Darden, I was even more impressed by the way you organized your talk at Duke University. Your speech—the way you presented it and what you covered in it—was outlined in a believable and logical manner. What you did worked. It worked very well."

It worked, I came to believe, because my personality complemented Jones's. He hated structure, and I liked it. He was free-flowing; I was organized. He was general; I was specific. He talked loose, and I talked tight. And that's why we worked together so successfully for the next two decades.

Kim Wood, a longtime Jones associate and Nautilus distributor, and NFL strength-training coach, said it this way: "Arthur had all these training *pearls* that he uncovered, created, and described in his unique, attention-getting manner. But for whatever reason, he couldn't, or wouldn't, pull them all together. Darden polished the pearls and provided the string."

More important, the Duke lecture gave me a structure through which I could do serious research. I could test, quantify, and refine the principles I'd outlined. And I could also write about what I learned; I went on to author more than three dozen books on high-intensity training, including the one in your hands.

CHAMPIONS BELIEVE IN

THE ADVANCED MUSCLE AND POWER BUILDING MAGAZINE

MUSCLE

BUILDER/POWER

25p

K 48632

OCTOBER / $1.00

Something New in BLASTING THE ARMS! —you better believe it!

Bob Birdsong's BIG 20-INCH ARM PROGRAM Sensational photos—what a routine!

An Incredible Expose...! THE NAUTILUS MACHINES ...Only Joe Weider gets Five Great Champs to tell the truth in personal interviews

Why is the CALIFORNIA BODYBUILDER SO UNIQUE? He's more Muscular...more Defined...wins more Titles...! Why? It's all inside!

Ken Waller says: SERGE NUBRET MUST BEAT ME FIRST! before he can hope to beat the King, Arnold Schwarzenegger

Arnold's Mind Blowing Routine to BUILD BROAD SHOULDERS! Arnold Schwarzenegger's powerfully illustrated work-out! It'll make you sweat, blast, torture your shoulders to grow—grow!—GROW! Are you man enough...?

What you didn't know about VITAMIN C How does it help and how does it hinder the bodybuilder? You must know!

POWERLIFTING ■ WEIGHTLIFTING ■ COMPLETE SHOW RE

PART II

HITS FROM THE PAST

Arnold Schwarzenegger appeared on the October 1973 cover of *Muscle Builder/Power* magazine, with a tagline near his chin that read: "An Incredible Exposé . . . ! THE NAUTILUS MACHINES." Jones later discovered that the primary interviews, between Joe Weider and five champions, were fictitious.

In 1980, the magazine was renamed *Muscle & Fitness*, and since then, Schwarzenegger has been on the cover more than 30 times. In March 2004, he became its executive editor.

Chapter 5

HOW HIT HUMBLED SCHWARZENEGGER

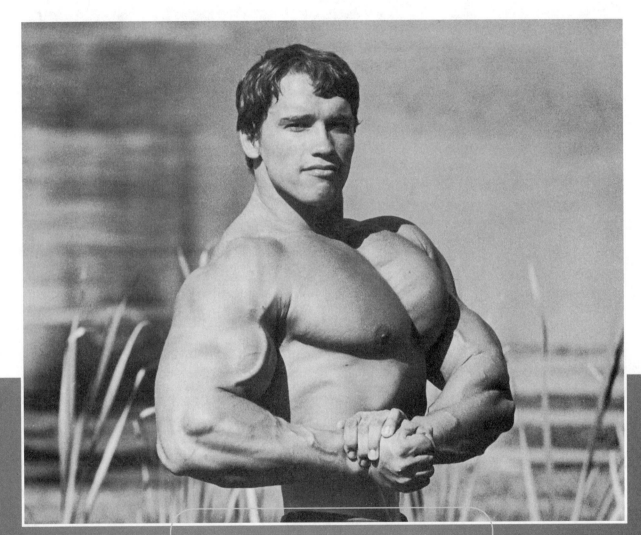

Arnold Schwarzenegger's massive chest is shown to advantage in this 1970 photo. Even though Schwarzenegger hasn't entered a physique contest since 1980—because of his action movies, media attention, and political ambitions—he's by far the most popular bodybuilder in the world today.

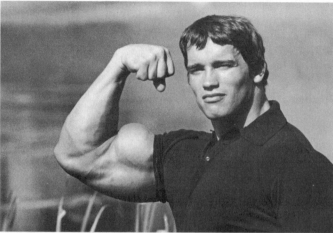

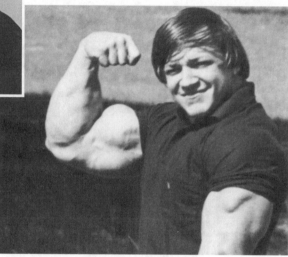

Interestingly, Jones measured Schwarzenegger's upper arm at 19½ inches and Viator's at 19⁵/₁₆ inches. He taped Viator's forearm at 15⁷/₁₆ inches and Schwarzenegger's at 13¹⁵/₁₆ inches.

When Arnold Schwarzenegger traveled to Florida in 1970 to train with Casey Viator, these separate photos were snapped on the first day in Arthur Jones's backyard. Schwarzenegger refused to take off his shirt and pose with Viator. Perhaps he was still a little upset from the drive over from the airport. Finally, he agreed to flex his arm for the camera.

BACK IN THE old days, when gyms were more like dungeons than the antiseptic, air-conditioned health clubs of today, lifters had a saying: "Train hard or go home." In other words, if you didn't like the atmosphere, or couldn't take the heat, or wouldn't attack the iron with the right attitude, then you might as well sign up for the exercise class at the recreation center. You weren't welcome in the weight room.

Even then, most guys who thought they were training hard were probably confusing amount of exercise with intensity. But definitions aside, the concept behind the saying was valid.

I visited a gym like this in 1966 in Dallas. The gym, called Hercules Health Club, was owned by

Jim Witt, a big, good-hearted, but tough-as-nails powerlifter. You had to walk up a flight of wooden stairs to get to the training area, which included a couple of raised lifting platforms, chalk boxes, Olympic bars, benches, and a bunch of handmade dumbbells in one corner. Along one wall were three mirrors, a wall chart of muscles, and a few autographed, framed pictures of champion lifters. On the opposing wall were half a dozen windows, all of which faced an alley and a brick-sided building. All the windows were open the day I visited, and I noticed that the screen on the window nearest the stairwell had been ripped apart and shredded.

I asked what had happened to the screen.

"A guy wasn't up to the workout I was putting

him through. So he took the quickest exit to the parking lot," Witt said. "It saved me some time, not having to escort him down all those stairs."

That's the way it was in hard-core gyms in those days. And Arthur Jones's training center was no different.

The Austrian Acorn

When Jones picked up Arnold Schwarzenegger at the Orlando International Airport in November 1970, he was expecting to meet a strong, silent type. Schwarzenegger had just won his first Mr. Olympia title at the age of 23, and Jones just presumed him to be a serious, hard-core, no-BS kind of guy.

Instead, he got a monologue for most of the 50-minute trip from the airport to Lake Helen. "For 30 minutes, all I hear is how big, strong, and great Arnold is, and it's difficult to understand him with this heavy Austrian accent," Jones said.

This was an unusual situation for Jones, who

was and is an aggressive monopolizer of conversation. Jones had hoped that when they got to the freeway—after a half-hour of start-stop driving on surface streets—the bodybuilder would relax and let Jones talk for a bit.

"But, no, he gets worse—he's more boisterous. He's sitting bolt upright in the seat, looking around like a male giraffe in heat and still shouting his gibberish. So, without saying anything, I calmly pull over on the right shoulder. Stop. Cut off the engine. Get out of the car and walk around to Arnold's side. Open his door, grab him by his shirt collar, jerk him out of the seat, stand him up, and look him right between the eyes. And yes, he's still talking, but it's more of whisper."

Jones explained, in a way only Jones could, that if the bodybuilder didn't shut up, he'd get his ass whipped by a man twice his age and half his size. Worse, it was going to happen at that moment, right there on the shoulder of Interstate 4.

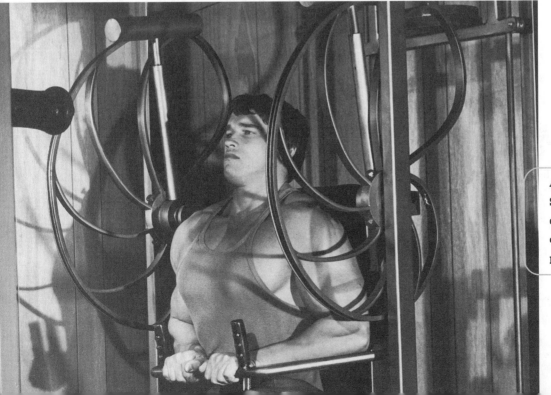

Arnold Schwarzenegger demonstrates an early Nautilus pullover machine.

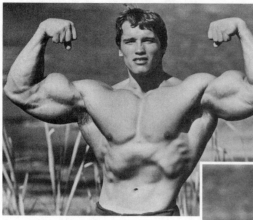

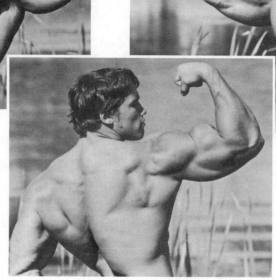

These photos of Schwarzenegger were taken after he had trained three times with Jones in Florida. Arnold had remarkable size, shape, and symmetry.

"Arnold stopped talking, grinned a bit, and nodded his head. Although I had difficulty comprehending his German, I guarantee he understood my English. And he knew I meant every word."

For the rest of the visit, Mr. Olympia showed proper consideration for Mr. Jones.

Arnold Watches and Writes Home

The next afternoon, Jones took Schwarzenegger to the Quonset hut at DeLand High School to watch Jones train Casey Viator. The best description of the workout was written by Schwarzenegger and published several months later in Joe Weider's *Muscle Builder/Power* magazine. The headline: "Arnold Invades the Viator Torture Chamber."

"Viator is a gym monster," he wrote (or, more accurately, a Weider editor wrote under Schwarzenegger's byline). "I never witnessed such ferocious, almost suicidal, training in my life. He kills the weights. He mangles the equipment. And most of all, he tortures himself to hysteria. Some day, he may have to be dragged from the gym in a straitjacket, and I'm not kidding. His main training principle is forced reps but not the kind I or any other star have the guts to do. I mean forced reps after the last normal rep has been forced out. He does forced reps until an observer could puke from horror.

"He switches from movement to movement. From apparatus to apparatus faster than you could take notes. He bangs away at each set until he can't muster another muscle twitch. He flushes each body part until the limb or area is paralyzed. This prime quality multiplied by dedication and madness no bodybuilder has ever approached. If I had to do this every day, I'd opt for a hernia, go back to Austria, and be a ski instructor."

What Schwarzenegger observed and described so well, he still failed to understand. There was no way Viator could have trained with that intensity every day. (Remember, Viator trained only six times in the 4 weeks prior to his Mr. America win.) And trying to do so, as Jones often said, would "kill a large male gorilla."

Loaded Magazines

From 1940 through 1970, Bob Hoffman and Joe Weider dominated the muscle-magazine business in the United States. Bob Hoffman published *Strength and Health* and *Muscular Development* magazines and sold food supplements and barbells from his offices in York, Pennsylvania. His chief claim to authenticity was his tenure as the Olympic weight-lifting coach. Joe Weider published *Muscle Builder/Power* magazine (which was later changed to *Muscle & Fitness*) in Union City, New Jersey, before he relocated to Los Angeles. Weider also sold barbells, training courses, and food supplements. Weider grew up in Montreal, Canada, and his background was little more than that of a dishwasher and short-order cook who had an interest in weight training and bodybuilding.

The April 6, 1970, issue of *Sports Illustrated* contained an article about Joe Weider entitled, "Be a Take Charge Blaster." Weider was identified as the man who "has replaced Charles Atlas as the world's leading builder of bodies." The article described Weider's use of a handful of champion bodybuilders throughout his magazine, as well as in the advertisements, which were "99 percent for Weider's products."

A picture of Schwarzenegger in a double-biceps pose adorned the first page of the article. Its caption read, "Weider student, Arnold Schwarzenegger, changes name to Arnold Strong." Schwarzenegger

changed his name at the request of a movie director, but used it for only one movie, *Hercules in New York,* which failed miserably at the box office when it came out in 1970.

But Jones had an alternate name-change theory:

The day before Schwarzenegger left Lake Helen to fly back to California, Jones was in the process of typing a photo release, which allowed Jones to use photos he had taken of the bodybuilder on Nautilus machines.

"When I finished typing the statement, I asked him how to spell his last name," Jones later told some of us. "Arnold gave me five different versions—all of them wrong." Finally, Arnold's buddy Franco Columbu had to tell him the correct letters to use.

"Arnold couldn't spell *Schwarzenegger,*" Jones smiled, "so he changed his name to Strong. He could spell that."

But let's return to the muscle world of the early 1970s.

Weider Joins the Battle

In 1971, Jones was no threat whatsoever to Weider, but Viator was a perfect specimen to add to the Master Blaster's stable of muscle stars. Weider used his magazine to invite Viator, who had always entered AAU competitions, to join his organization, the IFBB (International Federation of Bodybuilding). The 19-year-old Viator moved to Los Angeles briefly but soon returned to Florida to continue his work with Jones.

Viator's return to Lake Helen convinced Weider that Jones was a genuine competitor. He began a six-part series in his *Muscle Builder/Power* magazine criticizing Jones's Nautilus machines and his

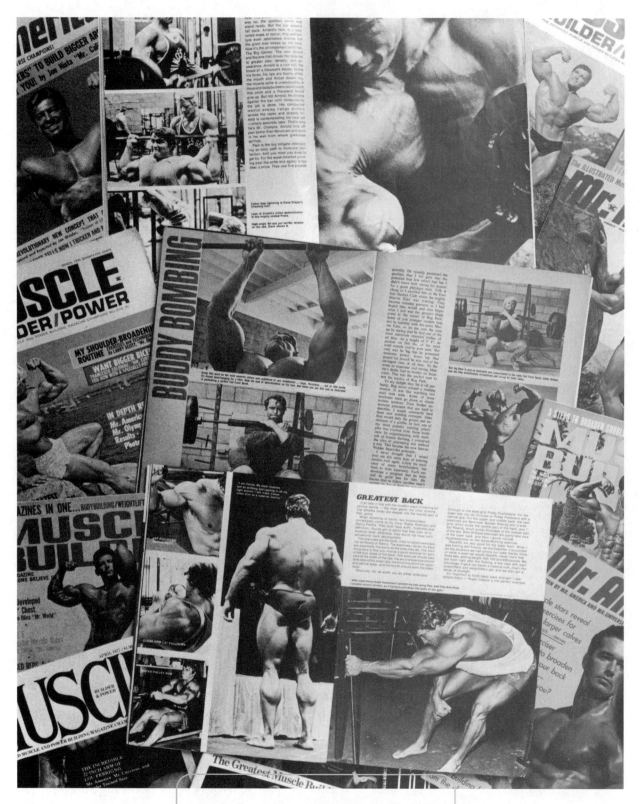

Joe Weider's muscle magazines of the 1970s
contained an assortment of blitzing, bombing,
multiple-set, and double-split routines.

Gaining Respect for Schwarzenegger

For a number of years, I was a member of the National Fitness Leaders Association, an honorary society of health and fitness leaders. (Because of federal budget constraints, the association was dissolved in 1996.) Each year, the group (from 75 to 100 strong) would assemble to discuss what we could do to improve the health of Americans. These meeting were always conducted with the cooperation of the President's Council on Physical Fitness and Sports. Usually in such meetings—where many well-known leaders, educators, and celebrities are present—very little gets accomplished. There are simply too many egos involved, and consensus of direction is almost impossible.

In 1990, however, things changed dramatically. Arnold Schwarzenegger was appointed, by the first President Bush, to be the director of the Council on Physical Fitness and Sports. Many of the group were alarmed and untrusting of Schwarzenegger (me included). But he came into his first meeting, challenged and united the leaders, and motivated all those in attendance. It was fascinating to watch the man in action. Furthermore, he not only talked a good game, he led by example. During the first year, he vowed to visit every state in the union (at his own expense) in the name of physical fitness. And he was true to his promise.

Schwarzenegger directed the President's Council for 2 years and accomplished more in those 2 years than all the previous directors had achieved combined. As a result, I gained a new respect for him. He may not ever be able to train in the true HIT style, but he can certainly push and motivate people to become more interested in physical fitness, particularly bodybuilding and strength training. I can now see why Schwarzenegger, in a special election held in 2003, was elected governor of California.

system of high-intensity training. The first part, in the October 1973 issue, was a lengthy interview with Schwarzenegger.

WEIDER: "Arnold, you went to Florida weighing a firm, muscular 226 pounds, and you spent 14 days training with Arthur Jones and Nautilus. What happened?"

SCHWARZENEGGER: "I came back looking terrible. You and others said I never looked so fat. And I lost three-quarters of an inch off my arms . . . and I really gave the biceps-curling machine a good, honest test."

Outright Hard Work—*Not!*

The truth, according to Jones, was that Schwarzenegger's workouts came nowhere close to "outright hard work," his definition of intensity. "I couldn't ever get him to work to failure, not even on one exercise. He'd strain and make terrible faces, but I can recognize the difference between faking failure and real failure. Arnold's was faked. But afterward, he'd talk like he'd had a great workout."

Viator had similar memories: "Arnold just couldn't get into the intensity part of it. He was used to going so far, backing off, resting, then doing another set. But our workouts were very, very, very intense, and there was no resting. He kept wanting to really get into it . . . and he seemed to be improving. But the last time Arnold tried to work out at the Quonset hut, in the middle of the session he crawled outside and spilled his guts on the grass. We didn't see him after that."

Both Jones and Viator calculated that Schwarzenegger was in Lake Helen less than a week, not 14 days.

But at least Schwarzenegger respected the old-timers' slogan. When he couldn't train hard, he went home.

Franco Takes Up Arms

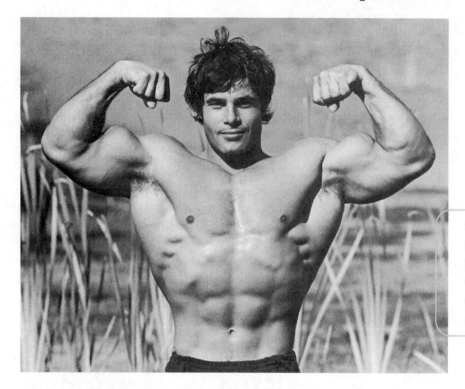

Franco Columbu, as he appeared the day before his November 24, 1970, workout. Columbu won the Mr. Olympia twice, in 1976 and 1981.

Another prominent bodybuilder, Franco Columbu, visited Lake Helen at the same time as his buddy Arnold Schwarzenegger. But Columbu, unlike his more famous friend, had an actual problem he needed to address.

"When I first saw Franco Columbu, at the 1969 Mr. Olympia contest in New York, his shoulder girdle literally dwarfed his arms," Arthur Jones said. "Later, Franco admitted to me that a lack of proportionate arm size was his greatest physical challenge."

Jones loaded his arms on the night of November 24, 1970. First, he accurately measured Columbu's arms cold, at right angles to the bone, on the first flex, using a paper-thin tape, which was then compared with a steel tape measurement.

He had the bodybuilder do 5 sets of Nautilus biceps curls and 5 sets of Nautilus triceps extensions, alternately, almost nonstop, with every set carried to momentary muscular failure. (Even though this was shockingly high volume by HIT standards, it was just a fourth of Columbu's normal 40-set arm routine.)

Next, he measured Columbu's pumped-up arms and found that each was $1\frac{5}{16}$ inches bigger than it had been cold. Jones said that was the biggest jump he'd ever seen in arm girth following a workout.

The next day, after the blood and other fluids had dissipated from his arms, Jones measured them again. Typically, arms will be equal to or smaller than their preworkout size. (With enough rest and proper nutrition, they'll start to grow after that.) But Columbu's were $\frac{3}{8}$ inch *bigger*.

As a side note, I should mention that Columbu, unlike his pal Schwarzenegger, had no problem tolerating the workouts. "He could take anything you'd throw at him, and he'd laugh about it afterward," said Larry Gilmore, who was present at some of the famous bodybuilders' workouts. "Arnold disliked being pushed. He refused to do the last 1 or 2 reps in each set. Arnold was 9 inches taller and weighed 50 pounds more than Franco, but Franco was stronger than Arnold on every exercise. Maybe that had something to do with it."

Chapter 6

THE ANTI-ARNOLD

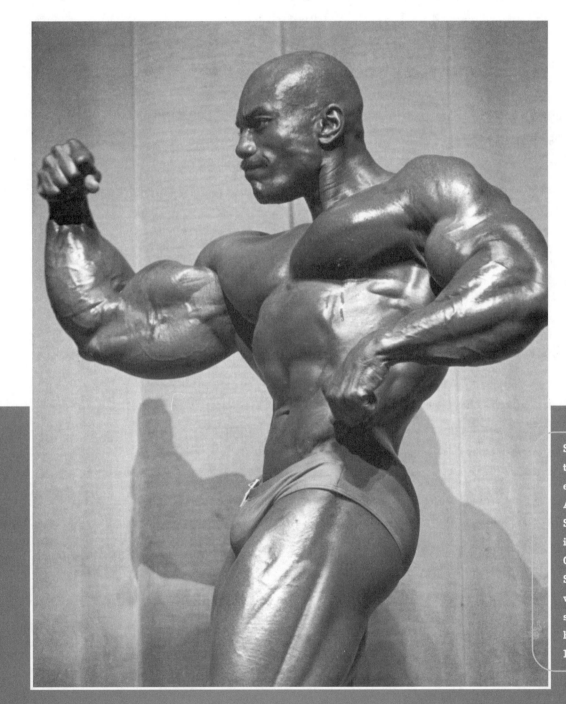

Sergio Oliva was the only man ever to defeat Arnold Schwarzenegger in the Mr. Olympia contest. Schwarzenegger won the title seven times, but he lost to Oliva in 1969.

I'VE SEEN ARNOLD Schwarzenegger and Sergio Oliva in their prime, on the stage posing and up close in normal clothes.

Schwarzenegger was 4 inches taller than Oliva and had better biceps peaks and chest height. Oliva had those massive upper arms and forearms, and when he expanded his chest and flared his lats, he had that dramatic difference between his waist and upper torso. I also thought Oliva was the better poser, moving with grace on stage while Schwarzenegger lumbered through his routine. Under competitive conditions, they were very different, but their strong and weak points cancelled each other out. I always thought it was a toss-up as to who had the better onstage physique.

Up close, however, in nonworkout clothes, Oliva was the decisive winner.

Bigger Than Dallas

It was dusk in Daytona Beach, Florida, in August 1971. Earlier in the day, I had watched as Arthur Jones put Oliva through a brief workout for his upper body. During the training session, Oliva's arms were the largest I'd ever seen on an individual—even larger than Casey Viator's.

That night, several friends and I were buying some ice cream on the Boardwalk, which overlooks the Atlantic Ocean. As we turned around with our ice-cream cones in our hands, there was Oliva, looking, as we used to say in Texas, "bigger than Dallas."

He had a green silk kimono draped over his shoulders and cinched at the waist, leaving the middle part of his chest and abdominals exposed. The bottom of the kimono barely covered his butt.

He had a thick gold chain around his neck, a large bracelet on one wrist, and a huge gold watch on the other. His arms from the mid-biceps down were uncovered. He also had on a small straw hat with a wide blue band, which included a couple of feathers on the side, and wore huarache sandals.

What surprised me most—other than the fact that anyone could pull off an outfit like that without looking completely ridiculous—was the size of his thighs. He told me they'd improved considerably since he started doing HIT routines with Jones. "And my mother in Cuba hears me scream every time I perform those last painful reps."

I watched his leg workout in the Quonset hut a couple of days later.

A Dead Man Walking

Oliva walked around nervously, looking at the floor and slowly shaking each leg, while two large football players put 480 pounds on the leg-press machine and adjusted the seat properly.

"Let's go, Sergio," Jones said. "I want 20 reps."

At 17 reps, Oliva looked whipped.

"Rest a few seconds in the lockout, and you'll be able to get 3 more reps," Jones said.

Oliva took five quick, short breaths and squeezed out 3 more repetitions.

Jones nodded to the football players, who literally picked Oliva up from the leg press and immediately helped him to the leg-extension machine. The goal, again, was 20 reps, this time with 200 pounds.

By the 10th repetition, Oliva was in obvious pain. Somehow, with Jones hurling insults about his manhood, he managed another 8 reps.

Once again, Jones signaled the football players,

Is Your Right Arm Smaller Than Your Left?

If you watch closely at a major bodybuilding championship, you'll notice something interesting: Almost every right-handed bodybuilder will have a left arm that's larger than his right. This is because the left arm of a right-handed person must work harder to perform its share of an equally divided workload. The left arm doesn't work more, and it doesn't work differently. It simply works with greater intensity. And it responds by growing larger than the right arm.

Let's say that you're right-handed. Your right arm, obviously, is better coordinated than your left. So your balance and muscular control are less efficient in your left arm. Therefore, your left arm works harder, and its response to this increased intensity is to grow larger.

In fact, in tests of strength that don't involve balance or muscular coordination, the left arm is almost always stronger than the right, as well as larger.

When this interesting fact is brought to the attention of most bodybuilders, their response usually is "Well, in that case, I'll do an extra set of curls and extensions with my right arm. Then it'll grow larger, too."

Which, of course, brings us back to the point of this book: To achieve growth, you need *harder* exercise, not more exercise.

---

and they pried Oliva from the leg extension and hurried him across the room to the squat stands. The bar had already been loaded to 420 pounds. Three weeks earlier, Jones told me, Oliva had performed a similar routine, but with less weight, and was unable to perform a single repetition with 400 pounds. "He'll do 420 pounds today and for at least a dozen repetitions," Jones said.

Oliva stepped back from the squat stands with 420 pounds on his shoulders and started the set. He strained so hard on the first rep that I didn't think he'd finish the second. But he did . . . somehow. The third rep looked equally brutal. Then he got into some sort of groove, and repetitions 4 through 10 seemed a bit easier than the initial ones, even though he was breathing and sweating like a steam engine. Repetition 11 went slow, and repetition 12 was very slow. True to Jones's prediction, Oliva failed on his 13th rep.

"Take the big plates off," Jones said to the spotters as they helped Oliva back up. "Okay Sergio, any

champion bodybuilder ought to be able to squat with 300 pounds."

Oliva looked at Jones as if he were having thoughts about dropping that barbell on Jones's neck.

Still, he responded with six perfect full squats with 300 pounds. Then he staggered to the stands, dumped the barbell, and collapsed on the floor.

I asked him if he was all right.

"He's all right," Jones said, as he finished jotting down some notes on Oliva's workout card. "He just needs a little rest before he works his upper body."

Jones allowed him to remain stretched out on the floor under the squat stands for exactly 20 minutes. Then he said to me, "Go get Sergio up."

I walked over to where Oliva was lying on his back. I knelt down and tapped him on the shoulder. No response. His body felt cold and clammy. "Arthur, he looks dead to me," I said.

Just then I noticed Oliva's left eye open. He smiled. "Arthur wouldn't let me die—at least not

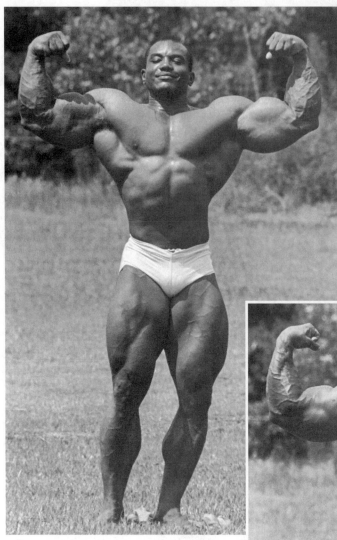

At a height of 5 feet 10 inches, Sergio Oliva weighed 233 pounds, and each of his arms measured cold was 20⅛ inches.

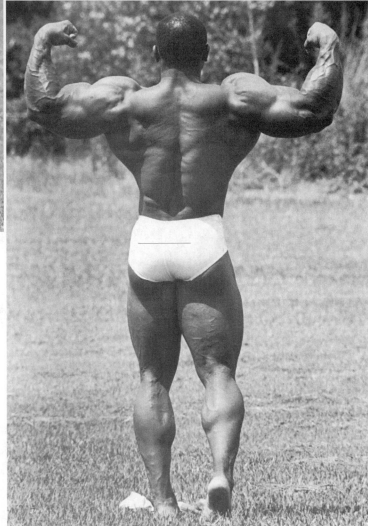

The awesome front and back double-arm biceps shots of Oliva, which were set up by Arthur Jones with a long lens in 1971. Oliva, according to Jones, is the only man who has ever had a muscular arm that was wider than his head was high.

until I've finished the workout. Here, help me get up."

In Praise of Freakish Muscle

Oliva's legs were large and muscular almost beyond belief, but few of his contemporaries talked about them. That's because his arms were, in Jones's words, beyond belief.

"Men with an IQ of 200 are freaks," Jones said. "Men over 7 feet tall are freaks. And in the same sense of the word, Sergio is a freak."

The photos of Oliva on the opposite page were taken after Jones had trained him for 3 consecutive weeks. Certainly, Oliva was well-developed before he had ever heard of Jones, HIT, and Nautilus. But you won't find a photograph of him taken before he trained with Jones that shows him with arms that are literally larger than his head.

That is, if you look at his flexed arms, you'll see that their height—measured from the peak of his biceps to the bottom of his triceps—is greater than the height of his face from chin to crown.

No one else in the history of bodybuilding, Jones believed, could make that claim.

His hard work (and, yes, steroid use) had a lot to do with that. But he also started off with once-in-a-generation genetic potential. Oliva had unusually long muscle bellies in his biceps, triceps, and forearm muscles. (A muscle belly ends where the tendon begins. So a long muscle belly means a short tendon. I'll explain this in much more detail in the next chapter.) As a result, his upper arms and forearms had more room to grow thicker and wider.

But Oliva was doubly blessed: He had those long muscle bellies throughout his major muscle groups, allowing him to achieve a very rare combination of size and symmetry. Some of the bodybuilders today are more massive, but I have yet to see another with arms as big as his head.

Chapter 7

NOT YOUR AVERAGE PLAIN-ZANE ARMS

For more than 15 years, Frank Zane's symmetry, posing ability, and finely defined midsection allowed him to defeat most of the heavier, more massive body-builders of his day.

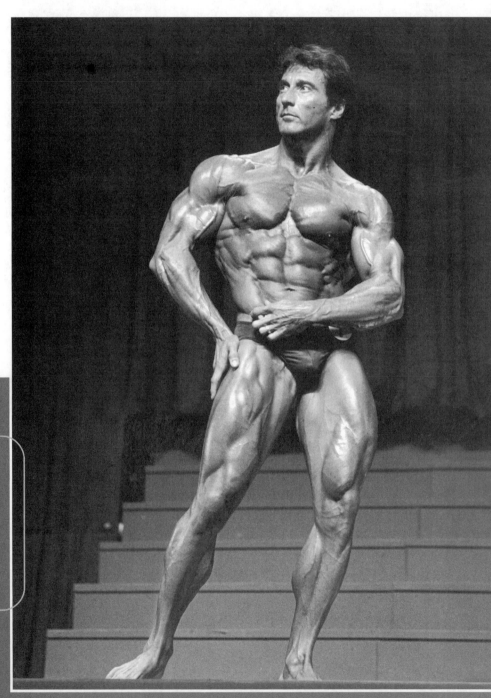

ARTHUR JONES WAS in his hotel room in London, England, the day before the 1971 NABBA (National Amateur Bodybuilders Association) Mr. Universe contest. There were a number of bodybuilders with him, including Frank Zane, who had won the amateur division the year before. Everyone was dressed in street clothes, and Jones noticed that Zane appeared particularly lean, light, and drawn, with highly defined cheekbones.

"Hey Frank, what do you weigh?" Jones asked.

"About 198 pounds," Zane said.

"You mean 168, don't you?"

"No, I weigh 198."

Jones offered to find a scale and settle the bet, but Zane quickly changed the subject, as Jones knew he would. After all, the room was filled with guys Zane was about to compete against, all of whom were quite a bit heavier.

Of course, size isn't everything in bodybuilding—or, at least, it wasn't back then. During his 15 years of competition, Zane's symmetry, attention to detail, and ability to pose allowed him to beat taller, bigger, and heavier bodybuilders—and beat them decisively—at the highest levels. He won Mr. Olympia three times (1977, 1978, 1979) and placed second three times (1974, 1976, 1982). His abdominals were considered by some to be the best in bodybuilding history.

More than anything, he gave the smaller, lighter man hope in bodybuilding. Still, like most guys who pick up a barbell, he couldn't help exaggerating. Lifters are notorious for rounding up, whether they're talking about their weight, their maximum bench press, or their arm size.

Armed and Dangerous

It was a late Tuesday afternoon in the winter of 1979. I was in my office at Nautilus Sports/Medical Industries, which overlooked the training floor. Because most people work out on a Monday-Wednesday-Friday schedule, the gym was empty, and I was ready to call it a day, lock up the place, and go home.

Just then, the door opened, and in walked Frank Zane and his wife, Christine. They were reorganizing their home gym in California and wanted to try some of the latest machines.

So we talked and tested equipment for a half-hour and then walked over to the main office to chat with Jones. We found him in his office, wearing his black, horn-rimmed glasses, reading the local newspaper. We'd barely gotten past the perfunctory greetings before Jones took out a pair of scissors and cut off a thin strip of newspaper an inch wide and a couple of feet long. Then he picked up a steel ruler and with a pencil started marking off the inches: first 0, then 15, 16, 17, 18, 19, and 20. I knew Jones was going to measure Zane's arm, but the bodybuilder suspected nothing. He and Christine chatted with Jones about his new leg-extension and leg-curl machines, and Jones answered their questions, as if nothing else were going on.

Jones then stood and walked around to the front of his desk, the strip of paper in hand. "What do you weigh now?" There was a pause that must have been 5 seconds . . . and I could tell that Frank was getting very uncomfortable. But then Jones refocused his eyes and said, ". . . Ell Darden?"

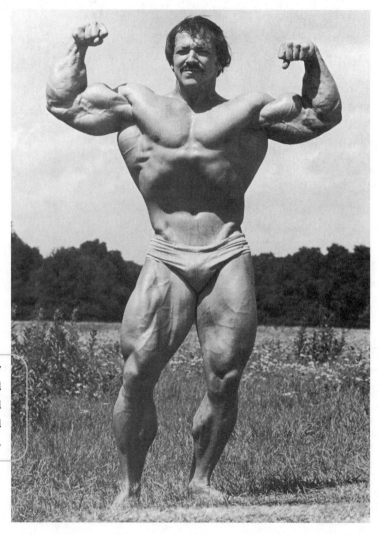

This is the way Casey Viator looked when Frank and Christine Zane visited Lake Helen in 1979.

Everyone in the room was surprised, me more than the others.

"Yesterday, I weighed 175½ pounds after my workout," I said.

Jones told me he wanted to measure my arm.

So I stood, pushed up my shirt sleeve, and contracted my left biceps as hard as I could. Seven years earlier, in my best shape ever at 195 pounds, Jones had measured my arm at 16¾ inches.

"That's 15¾ inches," Jones said. "Pretty good arm for a former bodybuilder."

Just then, Casey Viator walked into the room, almost as if on cue. (A quarter-century later, I'm pretty sure it wasn't planned that way.)

After a quick round of greetings, Jones said he wanted to tape Viator's arm, noting that he hadn't measured it in a couple of months.

Viator pushed up his sleeve, opened and closed his fist several times, and slowly contracted his right arm. The biceps rose so dramatically that it looked as if it would burst through his skin.

Jones wrapped the newspaper tape around

Viator's huge arm. "It's a shade over 19 inches, say 19¹⁄₁₆. Here, Frank, you and Christine stand up and have a look."

Viator's arm, for some reason, always looked even bigger when it was 6 inches from your face.

"Casey weighs 205 pounds, which is 13 pounds off of his best body weight of 218," Jones said. "When Casey won the Mr. America, his arm measured exactly 19⁵⁄₁₆ inches."

Then Jones put away his strip of newsprint, which took the tension out of the room. None of us wanted to see Zane put on the spot, least of all Frank and Christine. Besides, Jones had made his point. Everyone in the room, including Zane, knew his arm was bigger than mine, even though we both weighed about 175 pounds. And we all knew Zane's arm wasn't nearly as big as Viator's.

Length, Girth, and Mass

The demonstration gave Jones a chance to expound on one of his favorite topics: the advantage of having long muscles and short tendons. He drove the point home by having Viator contract his biceps, triceps, and forearms and then having me do the same. The difference was clear: My arm muscles were significantly shorter than Viator's.

(As a side note, Jones could always correlate a bodybuilder's body weight with his arm size—he could measure one and then accurately predict the other. He could do something similar with crocodiles, alligators, and rattlesnakes, correlating their head size with body length and body width, which is yet another example of Jones learning something in one field and then applying it to a completely different pursuit.)

Jones noted that Viator and I had very similar upper-arm bones. That is, we had about the same distance between our shoulder and elbow joints. But my biceps tendons were about an inch longer, which means the belly of my biceps muscle—the part that produces size—was about an inch shorter.

Then he had us straighten our arms and contract our triceps. "Casey's triceps muscle bellies run almost to his elbow tip. Ell's stop a good 3 inches from his elbow."

Jones brought out a yellow tablet and wrote these numbers:

6 inches and 9 inches

$1.5 \times 1.5 = 2.25$

$1.5 \times 1.5 \times 1.5 = 3.375$

The numbers showed that if Viator had a triceps length of 9 inches, versus my 6 inches, then his triceps were 1.5 times as long as mine. The square of those numbers shows that Viator had 2.25 times as much potential cross-sectional area. The cube of those numbers shows that Viator had 3.375 as much mass potential.

So if Viator and I trained in a similar manner, which of course we did, then he could expect approximately 3.375 times as much triceps size. (Nobody said life was fair.) In fact, that's why I got out of competitive bodybuilding when I did. I knew I'd gone as far as I could with my potential.

But Zane, as the reigning Mr. Olympia, was in a very different situation. He couldn't very well just quit. But that also wasn't Jones's point.

He next explained that having short triceps doesn't necessarily mean that all your muscles are short. He had observed differences between the muscles on the back of the body and those on the front, and from one muscle group to the next.

Zane asked if there was any way to lengthen a genetically short muscle—something many bodybuilders claim they can do with one exercise or another.

"No. Preacher-bench curls, contrary to what you read in the magazines, won't lengthen your biceps, and heavy barbell pullovers won't lengthen your triceps. The length of your biceps and triceps—any muscle group, for that matter—is 100 percent genetic. What you are born with is what you must live and die with."

Size Yourself Up

Let's begin by examining your biceps. Take off your shirt and hit a double-biceps pose in front of a mirror. Look closely at the inside elbow area of both arms. Now, pronate your hands (turn them away from your head), then supinate them (turn them toward your head). Notice that when you supinate your hands, your biceps get more peaked. That's because the primary function of your biceps is supination of the hand.

Go back to the double-biceps pose with your hands fully supinated. The bend in your arms, or the angle between the bones in your upper arms and forearms, should be 90 degrees. Look at the gap between your contracted biceps and elbow. How wide is that gap?

Before you measure it, relax your arms for a few minutes. While you're relaxing, do the following: Take your right hand and place your fingers across the crook of your left elbow. You should be able to feel the large tendon of the biceps as it crosses the front of the elbow joint and inserts into the radius bone of the forearm. In fact, as you gently contract your left biceps, dig your fingertips into the elbow

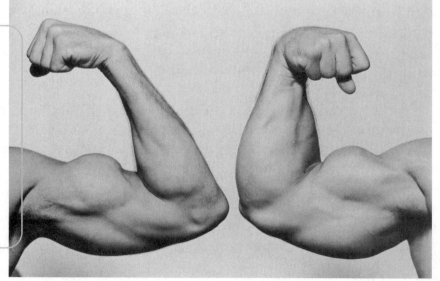

On the left is an above-average-length biceps muscle, and on the right is the long biceps muscle of Casey Viator. Notice the difference between the size of the elbow gaps and the mass of the biceps. Also, the forearm flexor muscles on the right arm are much longer and more massive.

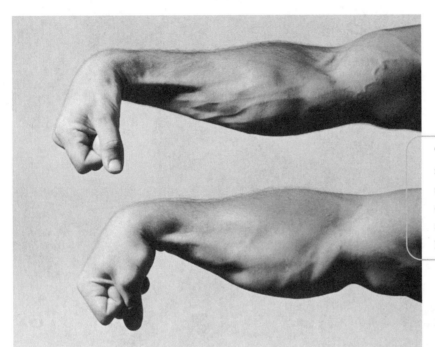

This photo compares the right forearms of the same two men. Examine closely the muscle length and the mass of the bottom forearm.

gap and get a good feel of the cablelike tendon. Follow the tendon up the arm until you feel where it merges into your biceps. Your goal is to determine the distance between the spot where your biceps meets the tendon and where the tendon crosses the elbow joint.

Hit the double-biceps pose once again. Make sure your hands are fully supinated and that the bend in your arms is 90 degrees. Have a friend measure with a ruler the distance between the inside of your elbow (look for the crease in the skin on the front side of your elbow) and the inside edge of your contracted biceps. Do it for both arms.

What do the resulting figures mean?

Although this is not an exact science by any means, my experience leads me to some rough estimates.

BICEPS POTENTIAL FOR BUILDING MASS

Distance between Elbow and Edge of Contracted Biceps	Biceps Length	Potential
½" or less	Long	Great
½"–1"	Above average	Good
1"–1½"	Average	Average
1½"–2"	Below average	Poor
2" or more	Short	Very minimal

The bodybuilders with the really massive arms all have a distance of ½ inch or less between their elbows and contracted biceps. In other words, their biceps have long muscle bellies, short tendons, and great potential.

Sergio Oliva, the man with the most massive arms I've ever seen, has biceps that are so long that there are no gaps between his elbows and

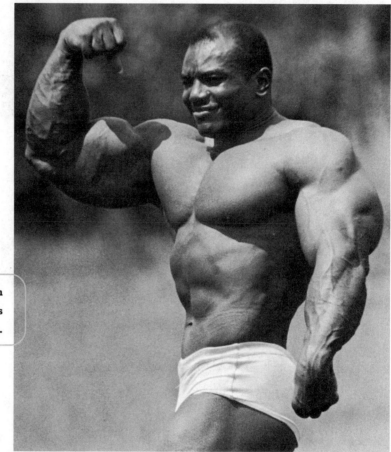

Check out the length of Sergio Oliva's biceps and triceps.

contracted biceps. That's right: zero inches.

Although no one questions the importance of well-developed biceps, the muscle that contributes the most to the mass of the upper arm is the triceps. But its length is harder to determine. The junction between the three heads of the triceps and their common tendon is more difficult to measure and evaluate.

All three heads of the triceps—lateral, long, and medial—attach to a large, flat tendon that runs across the back of the elbow and connects to the forearm bone.

Take off your shirt again and look in the mirror. Turn to your side. With your elbow straight and your arm by your side, contract your triceps. You should observe, if you are reasonably lean, a distinct horseshoe shape. The lateral head of your triceps forms the outside of the horseshoe, the long head forms the inside, the medial head lies beneath the long head, and the tendon occupies the flat space in the middle.

I've observed over many years that men with really massive triceps have less of a horseshoe shape. The flat space in the middle of the horseshoe is partially covered by the unusual length of the long head at the top. And the lateral and medial heads on the sides resemble upside-down soft-drink bottles. What's left of the tendon is about the size of a credit card rounded off at one end.

Sergio Oliva, for example, had no horseshoe shape at all to the back of his arms. Ditto for Casey Viator and Mike Mentzer.

Here's how to determine your triceps potential. With your elbow straight and your arm by your side, contract your triceps. Have a friend measure the distance from the tip of your elbow to the top of the inside of the horseshoe. In other words, you measure the longest portion of the flat tendon. Remember, the longer the tendon, the shorter the muscle, and vice versa.

Here are my rough guidelines for estimating your triceps potential.

TRICEPS POTENTIAL FOR BUILDING MASS

Distance between Elbow Tip and Top of Inside of Horseshoe	Triceps Length	Potential
3" or less	Long	Great
3"–4"	Above average	Good
4"–6"	Average	Average
6"–7"	Below average	Poor
7" or more	Short	Very minimal

You can still have massive triceps even if your long head is depressingly short—as long as your lateral and medial heads are long and thick. The triceps chart, therefore, is not as accurate as the biceps chart.

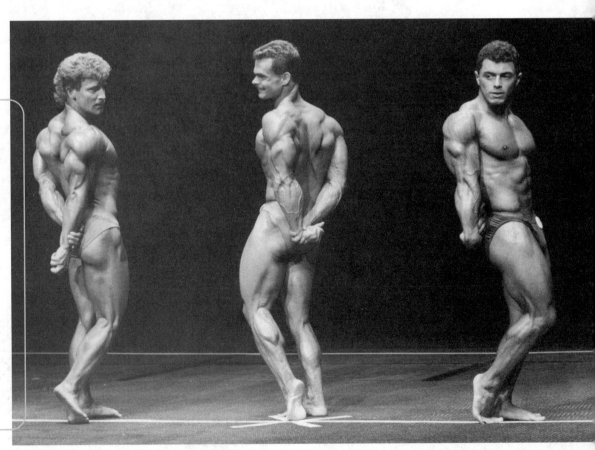

To determine your triceps potential, straighten your arm and contract your triceps (as shown), and then have someone measure the distance from the tip of your elbow to the top of the inside of the horseshoe. Compare your number to the chart above.

Chapter 8

MILITARY MUSCLE

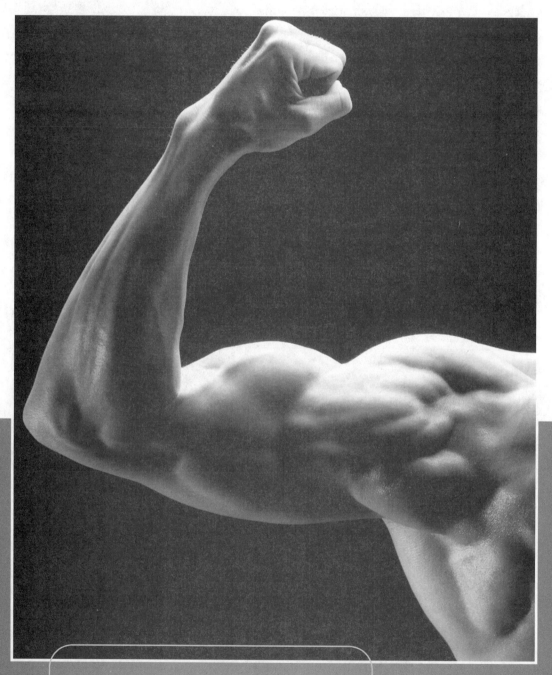

Physical strength is important to the armed forces.
That's one reason why the U.S. Military Academy at
West Point, New York, was the setting for a 6-week
HIT study in 1975.

"PHYSICAL EDUCATION IN the United States stinks. It's been a disastrous failure."

These were Arthur Jones's opening remarks when he addressed the Florida Physical Education Association's annual convention in Orlando in the fall of 1974. You better believe he got everyone's attention.

He didn't let up after that.

"If everyone in the United States realistically rated his or her lifetime physical-education experiences on a scale of from minus 10 to plus 10, the combined overall average would be something on the order of minus 4. Physical education activities have caused more harm than good."

The audience was quiet—no fidgeting or nervous whispering. Attendees were sitting upright and listening intently.

"If everyone in the United States today, at this very moment, stopped participating in any and all physical fitness activities, then the health of the nation would improve significantly in a matter of weeks. Why? Because people would stop being injured, and the average score would rise to something closer to zero."

Jones concluded his talk by noting that exercise, when it's performed correctly, should never cause an injury. Exercise should strengthen, improve, and enhance your body—and it will, if you don't destroy your body in the process of exercising.

Running to Nowhere

I should put all this in context: At the time of his lecture, the mid-1970s, the running craze was at its peak, and something like 80 percent of runners were being treated at orthopedic clinics throughout the United States. (Today, government statistics show that at least 20 million Americans each year suffer injuries that resulted from exercise, fitness, and sports activities and that require medical consultation.)

The leading running guru at that time was Kenneth Cooper, M.D., who had a couple of best-selling books, *Aerobics* (1968) and *The New Aerobics* (1970). Dr. Cooper believed that running was the best way to achieve cardiovascular endurance, and he advocated steady-state endurance activities as the core of every exerciser's workout program. He didn't have anything against occasional weight training for muscle strength, but he didn't have much use for it either.

Jones, of course, had a different take. He said that running was a limited, midrange activity. It would certainly work your heart and lungs, if the repetitive pounding didn't destroy your knees and other joints during the process. But running did almost nothing for strengthening most of your major muscles, and it decreased your flexibility.

High-intensity weight training, the kind Jones had been using, would not only strengthen your skeletal muscles but also involve your heart and lungs to a high degree and make your joints more flexible, without the pounding associated with running. The problem was that Jones didn't have any scientific research to support his contention. Poorly designed studies had been done in the past using barbells, but nothing had been attempted involving Nautilus machines and Jones's nonstop way of going from exercise to exercise.

Research and Education

To get the high-quality research he needed, Jones had to get the cooperation of the physical education department of a major university. And, unlike his study of Casey Viator at Colorado State University, he needed to do the research with many subjects, along with a control group. He had a few contacts at Ohio State, Georgia Tech, and Clemson, but those didn't show much promise.

Finally, Nick Orlando, the Nautilus distributor in New York, mentioned that he had just sold a line of Nautilus to the U.S. Military Academy at West Point. Orlando made a few calls, and soon he and Jones met with James A. Peterson, Ph.D., a professor in the physical education department. They agreed that Nautilus would do the funding and the training, and West Point would provide the subjects, testing, and statistical evaluations.

I was thrilled when Jones asked me to go to West Point in early 1975 to help supervise the study. I was already convinced that HIT was the best training system, and I'd worked with hundreds of people in Florida and Georgia who were experiencing similar results. Still, most coaches and athletes—to say nothing of the general population—did not see strength training as a viable way to develop strength, endurance, and flexibility in tandem. The idea that you had to develop these fitness components separately still prevailed.

The plan was to recruit West Point football players and divide them into two groups of 20. The study would last 6 weeks. One group would train the Nautilus way; the other group would train the traditional West Point way. Before-and-after measurements for strength, endurance, and flexibility would be performed, statistical tests

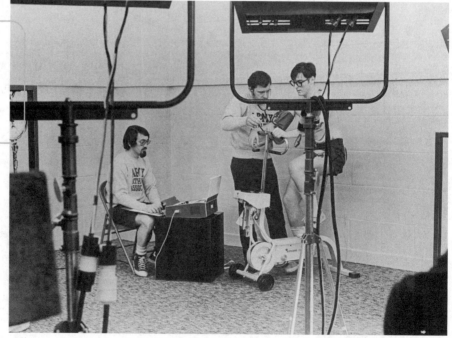

Dr. Don Franks (seated) and Dr. Larry Gettman conduct the pre- and post-cardiovascular tests on the two groups of West Point cadets.

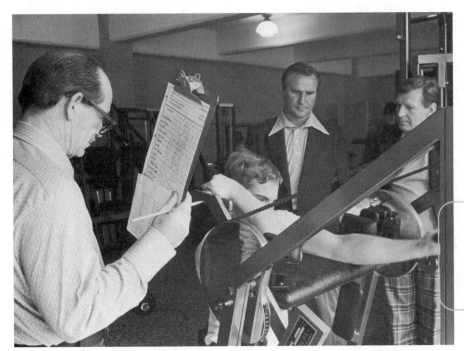

Arthur Jones supervises a cadet in the biceps-curl machine, as Coach Don Shula and Dr. Robert Nirschl observe.

applied, conclusions drawn, and the entire study reported.

Army's football coach, Homer Smith, didn't want his first-team football players involved, but we still had plenty of motivated second- and third-team players to use for the study. We also arranged to bring in two colleagues of Dr. Kenneth Cooper to conduct the cardiovascular-fitness tests. That would head off skepticism about whatever results we obtained.

Jones and I did the one-on-one training of the athletes, with an occasional assist from Tom Laputka and Nick Orlando. Each cadet was pushed to a maximum effort with one set of 8 to 12 repetitions; we increased resistance anytime he could complete 12 reps with good form. Each cadet did three workouts a week, and a workout usually included 12 or fewer exercises. We varied the work-

outs but kept precise records of every set performed. We even filmed some of the sessions.

Almost every cadet became nauseated at least once or twice during week 1. The workouts were brutal, unlike anything any of them had experienced. The cadets told us they were even more intense than their football camps and the various initiation rituals they underwent in military schools. Stories started spreading around the dormitories about the Nautilus torture chamber. Jones, of course, loved the idea of creating a mystique around his workouts and machines and instructed everyone in the study to clam up.

The Mystique Grows

It worked. Soon, cadets were dropping in to watch the workouts. So we shut and locked the doors and posted signs forbidding entry without authorization. That created even more interest.

After 3 weeks, the effects of the program were evident. The athletes using HIT were noticeably bigger, stronger, leaner, and more confident. Spring football practice was underway, and the Nautilus-trained guys were performing at a higher level than their coaches and teammates expected. Jones brought in Don Shula, coach of the Miami Dolphins, for a day. When Shula addressed the football team, he said that the Dolphins had used similar training in 1972, 1973, and 1974. Most of the players knew that the Dolphins had won the Super Bowl two of those years, and in case they didn't, it was hard to miss the championship rings on Shula's fingers.

After 4 weeks, we started an after-hours program so that some of the physical education faculty and athletic coaches could experience the training firsthand. Colonel Al Rushatz, the phys ed department's second in command, needed just three Jones-supervised workouts to realize that he'd misunderstood what Jones meant when he talked about "intensity." His skepticism started turning to amazement. Sergeant Dan Riley, the resident barbell instructor at West Point, was even open to being trained. Two track coaches started strength training, which was unheard of for them. Wives and sons of faculty members also fell in line.

Soon, everyone involved referred to our program as Project Total Conditioning. The Nautilus room was turning into a late-night fitness center, and the ghosts of West Point were howling in their sleep.

The sixth and final week of training was amazing. Jones and I were straining to come up with a new cycle or two to shock our trainees. They took everything we could throw at them, and though they didn't exactly smile afterward, they sure didn't buckle.

The Results Are In

Here are some of the results from the 6-week study. We ended up with 19 subjects in the experimental group (those doing HIT on Nautilus machines) and 16 in the control group (using free weights and standard training methods).

Muscular strength: This was the amount of weight a subject could handle for 10 repetitions with good form. After 17 workouts, the Nautilus group increased their strength by an average of 59 percent in each of 10 exercises. In other words, their strength increased about 10 percent per week per exercise . . . while they were participating in spring football.

The free-weight group, on average, didn't see any strength gains.

Cardiovascular endurance: Subjects were wired with a continuous EKG and blood pressure cuff and tested several different ways, including an all-out test on a stationary bicycle. They also did a 2-mile run.

The results were amazing. On every one of the tests that involved heart rate and blood pressure, the Nautilus group was significantly better than the control group. The HIT training caused the players to work more efficiently—in other words, at a lower heart rate—during all types of exertion. And on the 2-mile run, which wasn't monitored for heart rate, the HIT group reduced its average time by 88 seconds. The control group also did better, running the 2 miles faster by 20 seconds, on average.

Remember, both groups were also going through spring football practice, which helps explain why

Tackle *This*

Jim Hollingsworth was a defensive tackle for the Army football team, about 6 feet 3 inches tall and 230 pounds. Neither Arthur Jones nor I particularly liked to train him; he complained and talked back and wasn't a particularly hard worker.

But halfway through the program, something changed. He'd lost a few pounds of fat, gained a few pounds of muscle, and suddenly became one of our hardest-working cadets. His complaints and back talk became "yes sir," "no sir," and "I think I can get another rep, sir."

Here's what Hollingsworth did on the last day of the program in May 1975.

6:00 A.M.: Wake-up call.

6:30 A.M.: Breakfast.

8:00–9:30 A.M.: Test in Advanced Mathematics.

10:00 A.M.: Last Nautilus workout, consisting of squat machine, hip and back, leg curl, pullover, negative chinup, negative bench press, behind-the-neck pulldown, arm cross, negative dip, four-way neck, and shoulder shrug. Total training time: 17 minutes, 37 seconds.

Then he ran downstairs to the dressing room, where he took a quick, cold shower and got back into his gym clothes. Then he ran up two flights of stairs to the intramural boxing ring.

11:00 A.M.: Intramural boxing finals, heavyweight division. Hollingsworth won by a knockout in the first round.

Noon: Lunch at the mess hall.

1:15 P.M.: Report to football field house for taping and warmups.

3:00–6:00 P.M.: Annual spring football game. Hollingsworth suited up for the Gold team, made several key tackles, recovered a fumble, and was one of the most valuable players on the winning team.

Note: Jim Hollingsworth was a football letter winner at Army for 3 years and graduated with his class in 1978.

---

the average performance on the 2-mile run improved across the board. But spring practice doesn't explain why the HIT group reduced its running time so dramatically.

Joint flexibility: We measured flexibility in the trunk (both bending forward and backward) and in the shoulder joint. The Nautilus group improved on the three measures by an average of almost 11 percent. The average gain for the control group members was less than 1 percent.

New Believers

We'd shown the West Point instructors and coaches a way for their cadets to get more benefits in less time. In fact, several members of the West Point faculty went on to write books about high-intensity training.

Dan Riley not only wrote books, but he also became the strength coach at Pennsylvania State University in 1977—a much-higher-profile program, with athletes who were larger, stronger, and more gifted than those he instructed at West Point.

It wasn't long before Riley was one of the premier strength coaches in the United States, with many assistants working under his command. Penn State was in the hunt for the national championship almost every year.

Riley also wrote a monthly column for *Scholastic*

Coach, which circulated to high school coaches and trainers throughout the United States. He was soon in demand at coaching clinics, where he demonstrated his high-intensity techniques. Riley trained so many young interns and graduate assistants that today, there are dozens of strength coaches at major colleges, along with hundreds at high schools, who first worked for him.

Riley stayed at Penn State for 4 years, then got what he considered a great opportunity with the Washington Redskins.

The problem with jumping from a college environment—even a high-profile program such as Penn State's—to the NFL is that you quickly realize you have far less control. The athletes have more independence, and the head coaches and owners are less likely to stand behind their strength coaches and trust their judgment without hesitation.

When Riley interviewed with the Redskins in 1982, he told head coach Joe Gibbs, with no uncertainty, that he had to maintain control. Furthermore, the coaches had to understand what he was doing, which meant they too had to experience the nausea and light-headedness of high-intensity training. Gibbs liked Riley's boldness and assertiveness and hired him on the spot—with perks attached for playing in the championship games.

Gibbs and Riley had a great partnership. The Redskins won the Super Bowl in 1983, 1988, and 1992. After Joe Gibbs retired in 1993, Riley gradually lost some control as head coaches came and went. He got a chance in 2001 to establish a different NFL team's strength-training program from scratch, which he accepted. He's now the strength coach of the Houston Texans.

Riley has had—and still has—a tremendous influence on the strength-training practices of coaches and athletes throughout the United States. "Half the players in the NFL today train with some form of Arthur Jones's way," Riley told me recently. "They just don't speak of it in those terms."

And it all started with that West Point study, and the military muscle that it built, in 1975. It changed the way a lot of athletes trained.

Chapter 9

MENTORING THE MENTZERS

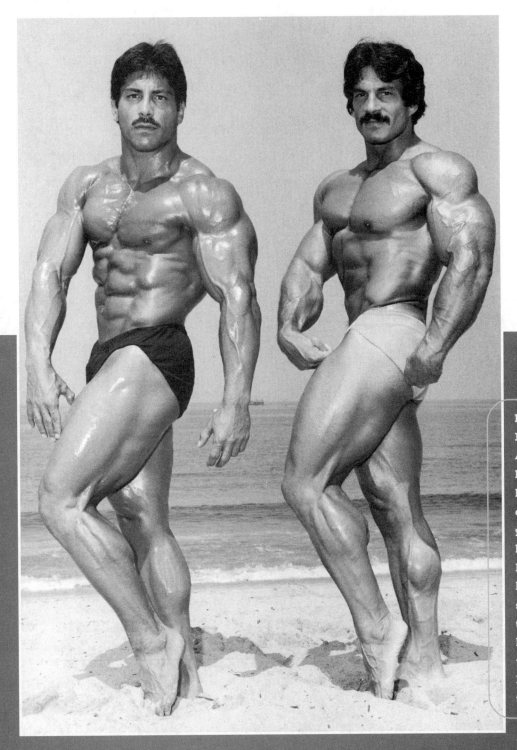

Ray Mentzer (left), 1979 AAU Mr. America, and Mike Mentzer, 1978 IFBB Mr. Universe, were examples of excellent genetics for bodybuilding. Both Ray and Mike had long muscles and short tendons throughout their bodies. This photo was taken at Venice Beach, California, in the summer of 1978.

WHEN ARTHUR JONES first saw Mike Mentzer in a bodybuilding competition, he thought that he noticed something familiar: Mentzer had long muscle bellies and short tendons, much like Casey Viator's. Mentzer finished 10th in that competition—the 1971 Mr. America—but Jones saw much greater potential.

I met Mentzer in 1973, when he first visited the Nautilus headquarters. I measured his arm at $17\frac{1}{8}$ inches, but with his long triceps heads, it was clear to us that he had a lot of room to grow. Indeed, Mentzer added 30 pounds of muscle to his physique and won the 1976 IFBB Mr. America and the 1978 IFBB Mr. Universe.

The next time we met was in 1978 in Los Angeles. Mentzer attended a presentation I gave at a Nautilus Fitness Center, then the next day took me to Joe Weider's headquarters in Woodland Hills. We worked out together at the Nautilus club and spent hours talking.

I didn't hear from Mentzer for several years, although I knew he was publishing books and articles about his training system, which he called "Heavy Duty." Then came the event that defined the rest of his life. He had spent all of 1980 preparing for the Mr. Olympia. He was the favorite to win and, when he got on stage with the others, he felt he was clearly the best bodybuilder that night. History shows that Arnold Schwarzenegger came out of retirement to win the 1980 Mr. Olympia, but many who were there agreed that Mentzer should've won, or at least placed higher than fifth.

Mentzer, by all reports, remained bitter about that loss for the rest of his life.

I next heard from him in 1981, when he asked me to write a series of articles for a new bodybuilding magazine he was starting. (In the wake of the Mr. Olympia loss, he'd quit competitive bodybuilding and cut off ties with the Weiders.) The magazine never got off the ground, although Mentzer did

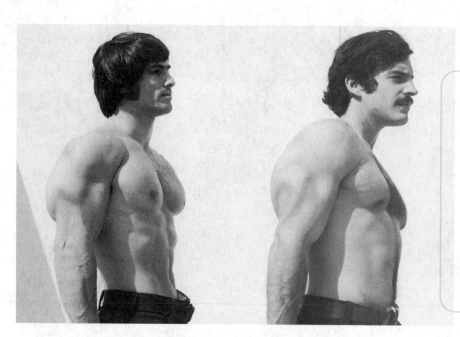

A 1973 photo of Richard Baldwin (left) and Mike Mentzer reveals that both had an arm size of $17\frac{1}{8}$ inches. Check out the extra thickness that Mentzer had near his elbow owing to longer triceps muscles, which allowed him to add another $1\frac{1}{2}$ inches to his arm circumference.

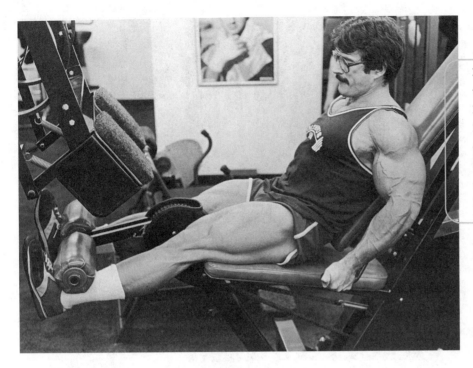

Mike Mentzer going through a HIT session in Los Angeles in 1978. Mentzer demonstrated great strength and was close to using the entire weight stack on each Nautilus machine.

write a foreword for my best-selling *Nautilus Bodybuilding Book,* which was published in 1982.

A Welcoming Workout

Mike and his brother, Ray, came to Lake Helen on January 5, 1983. Ray, 2 years younger than Mike, had never met Jones. In fact, all Ray could talk about that day was getting Jones to put them through a workout. After giving them a tour of his new video studio, Jones decided to *please* Ray—which was sort of like that old saying, "be careful of what you ask for; it just may come true!"

Ray Mentzer had won the 1979 AAU Mr. America at 5 feet 10 inches and 210 pounds. Now he was a good deal heavier at 253 pounds—massive, in fact—with an arm that measured 19¾ inches. He wasn't ripped by any means, but he wasn't fat either.

Jones started Ray with 385 pounds on the duo-

squat machine, in which you alternate legs on each repetition. After 8 slow, smooth reps with each leg, Ray was breathing like a freight train. But he continued at his deliberate pace, with Jones spurring him on, until he failed with his left leg on the 16th repetition.

Ray went back to work after Jones reduced the weight to 310 pounds. He huffed and puffed his way through 6 more repetitions with each leg.

"Damn, that's all I can do," he said to Jones. His face reinforced his words: He had bought it for the day.

"The hell you say," Jones said. "You came here to work, and you still can. Get ready."

With 85 pounds on the machine and a movement-restraining bar in place, Ray worked one leg against the other for another 30 seconds.

Ray's face contorted in pain. He screamed as he rolled out of the machine and collapsed on the floor.

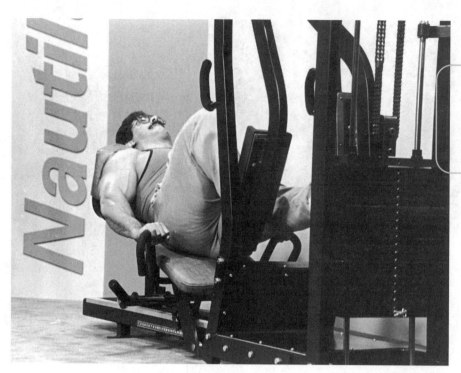

Ray Mentzer pushes through a hard set with the entire weight stack (500 pounds) on the duo-squat machine.

His legs resembled two vibrating machines twitching in unison as his body furiously pumped blood into his extremities.

Jones waited precisely 1 minute, then gestured to his assistants. "Help him get on his feet." The men pulled Ray from the floor; his face remained in a grimace. They measured his pulse rate at an astonishing 204 beats per minute, a full 60 seconds after he'd finished the exercise.

This was one of the biggest pumps I'd ever seen. Jones estimated conservatively that Ray's thighs had expanded by at least 2 inches. They were so swollen that Ray couldn't remove his sweatpants.

"Rest a few more minutes," Jones said. Ray took the offer like a whipped dog given a reprieve. But it didn't last long. "Up. Let's go."

Jones pushed Ray through seven additional exercises: lower back, chin, dip, pullover, pulldown, arm cross, and decline press. When he was finished, we measured his pulse rate again. This time it was 190 beats per minute.

"Damn it, Arthur, you almost did me in," Ray said.

Jones ignored him. "Try this program for the next 6 weeks," he said. "You do one set to failure of eight exercises, repeated only twice a week. I guarantee your body will respond. Cut your calories slightly to eliminate your excessive body fat." He studied Ray, who was still twisted up in pain. "Okay?"

"Okay, okay," Ray said. "I won't like it, but I'll do it."

"No one asked you to like it."

As Ray went off to the showers, he looked like the biggest kid in the neighborhood who'd just lost a street fight to someone half his size. When he was out of sight, Jones grinned. He knew a convert when he saw one.

Altered Seams

The Mentzer brothers flew back to California the next day. Ray continued his workouts, as Jones had instructed, and returned to Florida on February 21, 1983. He looked like a new man, 7 pounds heavier but much leaner.

Jones studied him carefully. "You stick with that program?" I knew the question was rhetorical; he wanted to gauge Ray's attitude more than anything.

"Like clockwork. Twice a week for 6 weeks." Then he told Jones that he'd needed to have his pants altered twice in the 6 weeks. The thighs had to be taken out, and the waist taken in.

Jones pretended to be unimpressed. "Let's see what your arm measures."

Ray rolled up his sleeve and contracted his biceps. Jones made the measurement, and his face brightened for the first time. "Now, pay attention," he said. "This shows what serious, no-nonsense

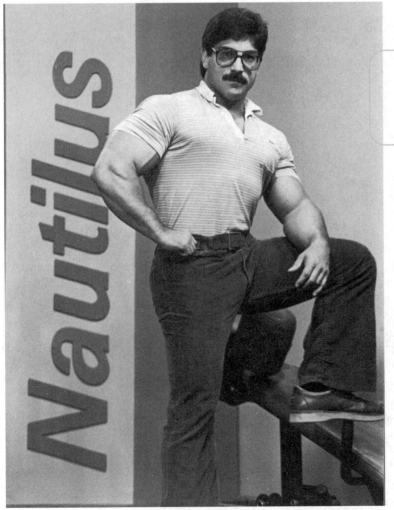

Ray Mentzer in fairly lean condition at a body weight of 250 pounds.

training can produce. It's 20⅛ inches. That ⅜ inch more than it was. And it looks like you've added at least 15 pounds of muscle."

The next day, Jones offered jobs to both Mentzers, and they accepted. And, to make things even better for me, Jones hired my old friend Boyer Coe, Mr. America 1969, at about that same time.

The Lost Boys

Jones had a habit of painting pictures of the future that were grandiose and motivating. But the many small steps that were necessary to get from here to there were left to his employees. Those employees, however, often found it tough to move forward without Jones's direction. The boss was involved in so many different projects at once that you never knew when he was going to give you feedback on your assignment. You had to be a self-starter to work effectively for Jones, and you had to be able to handle criticism—which proved to be a big problem with the Mentzers. Here's what happened.

Jones now had three well-known bodybuilders on his payroll, none of whom was in tip-top shape.

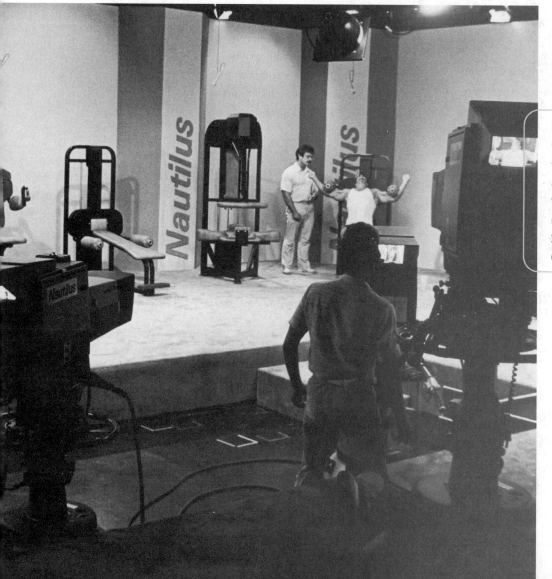

Eighteen complete workouts were videotaped of Boyer Coe at the Nautilus Television Studios in the spring of 1983. Here, Mike Mentzer monitors Coe on a chest exercise.

His initial plan was that each one would be trained intensely for 6 weeks in the Nautilus video studio, with cameras recording every repetition of every exercise of every workout. All the video would be edited and packaged into a body-transformation series featuring Coe and the Mentzers.

Coe volunteered to be trained first. Jones planned the routines, and he put Coe through his three-times-per-week workouts, with Mike or Ray stepping in when he couldn't make it into the studio.

The idea was simple: The cameras would roll. The trainer and trainee would walk into the room, introduce the routine, start the workout on the first exercise, keep the cameras rolling throughout the entire workout, summarize at the end, and walk off the set. No stops. No restarts.

But the execution wasn't simple at all. The first two or three workouts seemed awkward and stagy. Getting Coe, Jones, multiple video cameras, and all the lights in harmony was harder than anyone anticipated. Sometimes Coe or Jones looked in the wrong direction. The cameramen weren't always quick enough to capture the action. Coe didn't anticipate the extra heat generated by the studio lights, so he had to rest longer than expected between some exercises.

Things smoothed out somewhat during the second and third weeks of shooting. But then Jones had to travel for a week, and Mike and Ray stepped in to train Coe on camera. Mike couldn't get the hang of what he was trying to do at first. Ray looked awkward on camera and had to change shirts several times to blend in better with the surroundings. By that time, Coe was getting frustrated. The workout

was postponed until the following day . . . when a thunderstorm caused a power failure, leading to even more delays.

When Jones returned, there were more important things that needed his attention. I think he hoped Mike or Ray would take charge. But it didn't work out that way. Mike wanted Coe to try shorter routines. Ray thought longer workouts might be more effective, at least for a while. Coe stayed with the previous routine and sometimes ended up training himself.

To his credit, he never missed a workout. But just about everyone else was regularly testy, tardy, or delinquent. The workouts limped on, and little progress was made. The official end point kept changing, until the project finally dissolved. Coe started training with a friend in Daytona Beach after working hours. Mike and Ray sometimes worked out in the video studio but not when any cameras were rolling (which was a good thing; you wouldn't describe their workouts as superb examples of high-intensity training).

I tried to remotivate the guys by getting them to commit to appear in *The Nautilus Advanced Bodybuilding Book,* which I planned to write that summer and have photographed in October 1983. That would give everyone a summer's worth of training to get into good shape. All three agreed to help with the book and seemed sincerely interested.

As the summer progressed, however, I kept hearing that Mike and Ray were restless. Neither seemed able to find things around the video studios to keep them busy. We often found the brothers with their shirts off enjoying a long lunch break in the sun. That didn't go over well with

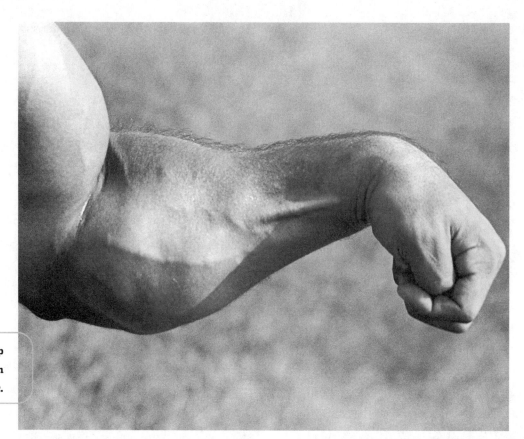

A close-up
of the forearm
of Ray Mentzer.

some of their colleagues. (Coe, on the other hand, was a natural, working hard on a number of Nautilus projects.)

The Short Goodbye

A turning point came one morning in early September. Jones came through the video studios with a group of medical and rehabilitation professionals. The largest studio was set up for a Nautilus seminar, featuring the new lower-back machine. Jones liked to spontaneously call upon employees to demonstrate exercises. The bodybuilders on his payroll were his favorite demonstrators, and Ray Mentzer, being the biggest, was his favorite of the

three. The Mentzers were in the studio at the time, so Jones waved Ray over and told him to show his guests how it worked.

"No," Ray said, without hesitation.

I don't think Jones heard him, because he never missed a beat in his description of the machine's qualities. But after a minute, he realized Ray hadn't followed his order. He turned around and said, louder than before, "Ray, where are you?"

"I'm right here, and I'm not getting up," Ray said, matching Jones's volume. Everyone in the room heard him this time.

Jones gave Ray a stare that would pierce armor, then waved to Mike, who hurried to the stage and demonstrated the machine for Jones's guests. When he finished, Jones led the group to another part of the facility.

Ray told a few people afterward that his back was still sore from a similar demonstration several days earlier, and he didn't want to risk hurting himself. But it didn't matter; he was fired and escorted off the property by the end of the day. Mike Mentzer was given the option to leave or stay. He at first chose to stay but 2 weeks later was gone.

The Bitter End

The Mentzers moved back to California. Mike finally got the backing he needed to start a new magazine, *Workout for Fitness,* which debuted in December 1984. I wrote a series of articles for him, but the magazine folded after nine issues. Ray worked briefly in a rehab clinic, which specialized in the use of Jones's lower-back machine, before relocating for several years to Australia.

Over the years, I heard stories about the Mentzers' battles with depression. Their behavior sometimes veered toward the surreal. Here's a story Jones told me, which took place in 1994:

Jones owned a ranch (which included his large array of elephants, crocodiles, alligators, snakes, a gorilla, a convention center, and an airstrip) in Ocala, Florida, that had a guard positioned at the front gate. One day, he got a call from the guard, who said there was a man in a taxi at the front gate who claimed to be Jones's son, Mike Mentzer. The cab fare from Orlando was $75, and the driver wanted payment now. Jones told the guard to stall the cab while he called the sheriff.

But the backstory is actually weirder than that. A mutual friend had recently warned Jones that Mike at times believed that Arthur Jones was the true God, and that he, Mike, was the son of God.

Mike continued publishing articles about "Heavy Duty" training. Toward the end, he prescribed routines that were so brief that only the most advanced and overtrained could hope to get results from them. I always liked Mike, but I didn't know what to think of him. In particular, I wondered how much true passion for training he had left in him. We talked seriously about bodybuilding only a few times, and that was mostly before he was employed by Nautilus. I watched him go through a true HIT workout, where he handled almost the entire weight stack on each Nautilus machine, in Los Angeles in 1978. But he never came into my office to talk about training during the entire 6 months we worked together in Florida. Not once! And I never saw him train hard in Lake Helen.

He died of a heart attack on June 10, 2001, at the age of 49.

Ray, on the other hand, enjoyed talking about exercise and could really get into the intensity factor. I put Ray through many workouts in Lake Helen; he and Casey Viator were the strongest men I ever trained. Ray died of a heart attack on June 12, 2001. He was 47.

Heart disease, I later learned, was prevalent in the Mentzer family tree.

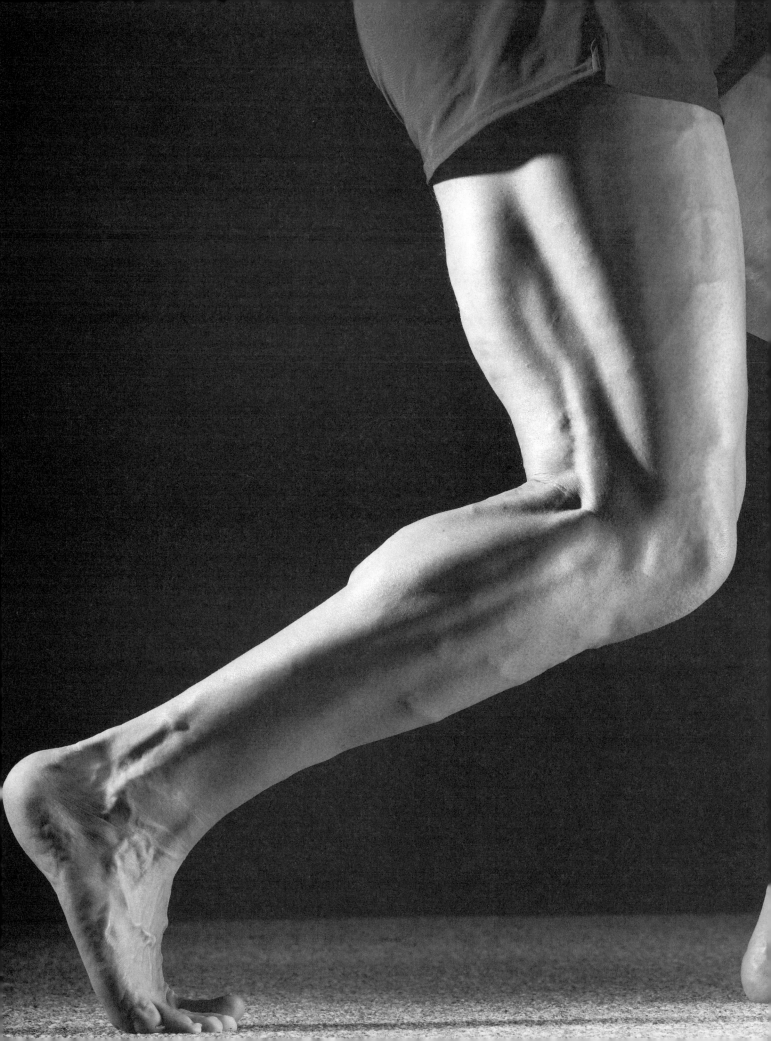

PART III

HIT PRINCIPLES, EXERCISES, AND ROUTINES

HIT is grounded in the concept that working the lower body takes precedence over the upper body.

Chapter 10

INTENSITY, FORM, AND PROGRESSION: GETTING YOUR PRIORITIES STRAIGHT

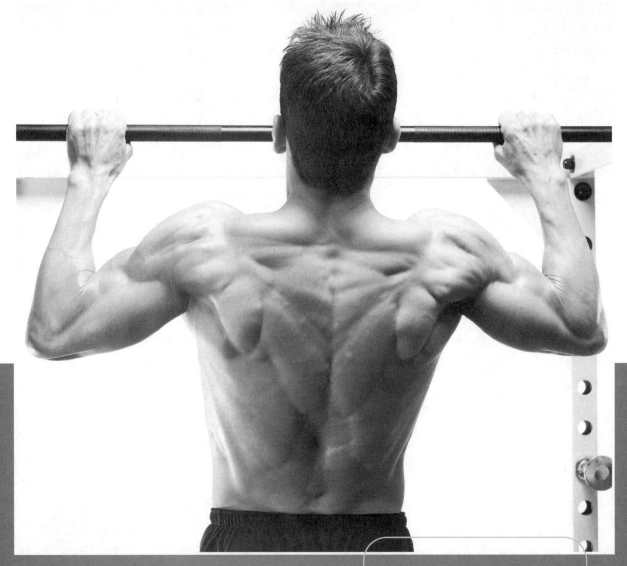

All chinning exercises demand intense muscular contractions and keen devotion to proper form.

I CAN SUMMARIZE HIT in nine words:

"Do as many repetitions as possible . . . in good form."

And yet, I'll be the first to admit that it's easier to describe than to do. Most of the trainees I've worked with over the past 30 years either didn't train hard at first or had pitiful form. Some had the worst of both worlds—little intensity *and* poor technique. Very few had both the intensity and the form. And only a small subset of those could maintain those qualities throughout their entire workout.

Yet, after 2 weeks of consistent instruction, the vast majority of these people could be guided or pushed through a HIT routine without losing their form. Thus, the primary goal of this chapter is to cover all the necessary points for putting maximum intensity into your training, as well as showing clear examples of the precise form for each repetition. I'll also discuss the best repetition range and progression schedule for your goals.

Intensity

Remember the "outright hard work" example from chapter 1? It provides a nice illustration of intensity but isn't a good example of proper form, at least not after the sixth or seventh repetition. Proper form requires consistency. Proper intensity requires a dogged determination to work through a certain amount of muscular pain to achieve every possible repetition.

That last phrase—"every possible repetition"— is what separates HIT from the standard "three sets of 8" or "three sets of 10" program. The HIT philosophy says you're much better off performing only

one set, but that one set must be carried to momentary muscular failure. If you stop at an arbitrary repetition—like number 8, number 10—and you could've done another, then you haven't worked hard enough.

Always do as many repetitions as you can, and then try one more.

Why you're better off with only one set is best understood by examining a number of critical factors.

Momentary muscular failure. Failure typically occurs when you can't continue the positive movement—the lifting portion—despite your best effort. After several seconds of trying to push or pull the resistance, you lower the resistance under control and stop the exercise.

Besides your positive strength, you also have a negative level, which can be worked to failure. I'll talk about negative training in chapter 15. And there's a type of failure that entails your lifting and lowering form, which I'll explain later in this chapter.

Strength inroad. Most of the time, you want to perform HIT sets with a 20 percent inroad into your starting level of strength. Here's what I mean by that: Let's say that you could do 1 repetition with 100 pounds on a leg-extension machine. A second repetition would be impossible. That means 100 pounds is your starting level of strength in the leg extension.

If you reduce the weight by 20 percent, you work with 80 pounds. That feels easy at first. But with each repetition, you make a deeper inroad into your starting level of strength. By the 10th repetition, your temporary level of strength is 81 pounds—just enough to lift the 80 pounds. You fail on the 11th repetition.

Thus, after 10 repetitions with 80 pounds on the leg-extension machine, you've reduced your starting level of strength to 79 pounds or less. You made at least a 21 percent inroad into your starting level of strength.

A 20 percent inroad is a good place to start, although you may find you do better with more or less weight. So in the leg-extension example, you might find you can do too many repetitions with 80 pounds and would get a better set with 85. That's a 15 percent inroad. Others may not get to 10 reps with 80 pounds and would perform a better set with 75, which is a 25 percent inroad.

Recovery ability. This describes the wide array of chemical reactions that must occur inside your body for your system to compensate from the stress of the workout and get you back to your previous level of size and strength. Your goal, of course, is to *supercompensate* and make adaptations to the workout that allow you to grow bigger and stronger. I'll get into the recovery issue in more depth in chapter 12, but here's what I want you to understand right now.

Your recovery ability does not increase in proportion to your ability to get stronger.

What this means is that as you get stronger, you must do less overall exercise. Because this is the opposite of how most lifters go about things, it's important to understand this concept from the start.

Less training. Ever try sprinting as fast as you can for a quarter of a mile, which is one time around a typical high school track? You'll be lucky to make even 300 yards at an all-out pace. In fact, perhaps only one man, Olympic champion Michael Johnson,

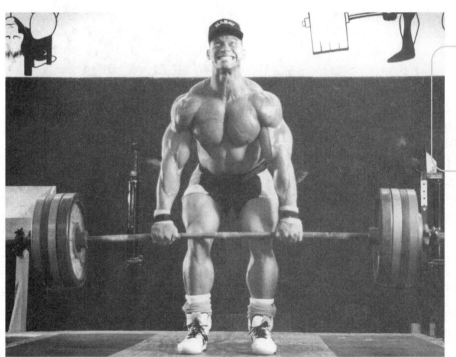

I personally trained
Keith Whitley, of Dallas,
for 6 weeks in 1990. The
stiff-legged deadlift was
one of Keith's basic
exercises.

Body of Evidence

Over the past 30 years, more than 40 studies have compared the strength-building effects of one set with those of two and three sets. Some research favored two or three sets, and some showed that one set was superior, but the vast majority of the studies revealed no significant differences between doing one set and doing multiple sets. They were all equally effective.

If that were truly the case, then one set wins simply because it requires less time. But of course, for all the across-the-board comparisons to make sense, all the studies would have had to apply a similar repetition protocol (which they didn't) and define failure identically (which they didn't).

So let's look at the theoretical reason that one set should work just as well as multiple sets.

Muscle-fiber recruitment. A muscle group is composed of thousands and thousands of individual fibers. These fibers work together, of course, but are also programmed to fatigue at different rates. That's why they're classified as slow, intermediate, or fast.

During a set of an exercise, the slow-twitch (type I) fibers are activated first. They are joined by the fast-twitch (type IIa) fibers, which have much less endurance than that of type I. As the type IIa fast-twitch fibers fatigue, they are replaced by the type IIb fast-twitch fibers, which will have even less endurance. When the type IIb fibers tire, the muscle is no longer able to finish the repetition, and the set must be stopped. There's definitely an ordering to the recruitment of muscle fibers during a set. And that ordering is genetic and not subject to change.

What happens if, after several minutes of rest, you perform a second set? Are different fibers involved? No. The same muscle fibers applied in the first set are again recruited in the same order during the second set. In other words, the stimulus is identical for one set, two sets, or even 10 sets. If you can stimulate maximum growth from one set—which you can—a second set merely uses up some of your valuable recovery ability. As a result, muscular growth is limited.

Animal examples. Need more proof of the value of intense, brief exercise? The next time you're at a large zoo, take a close look at the biggest male lion and the largest male gorilla. According to Arthur Jones, an adult male lion can get over a 10-foot-high fence with a 500-pound cow in his mouth. A mature 400- to 500-pound gorilla can perform a one-armed chinup so easily that he appears to weigh nothing.

A wrist that measures more than 8 inches on a man is huge, yet a 400-pound gorilla that Jones owned for many years had wrists that each measured more than 13 inches. The gorilla's neck, which in my opinion was his most impressive body part, stretched the tape to 33 inches.

Yet, according to Jones, lions and gorillas, even in the wild, perform almost no hard physical activity. But when they do work, they go at it with 100 percent intensity. The activity is hard, brief, and infrequent. Here's how Jones once put it: "I suspect that if you exercised a lion or a gorilla as much as many bodybuilders train, you would probably kill them, and it is certainly obvious that they do not need that much exercise. Neither do you; and even if you can stand it, it does not follow that you need it."

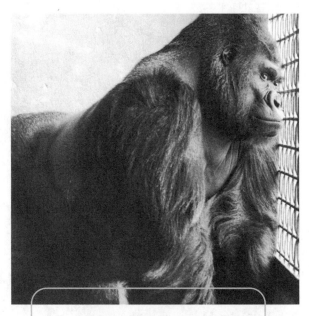

For a number of years, Arthur Jones owned a 400-pound gorilla that had 13-inch wrists and a 33-inch neck.

has actually been able to sprint a quarter-mile (400 meters), and that was during his world-record performance in the 1996 Olympic Games in Atlanta.

Going to failure on an exercise is similar to sprinting as far as you can. A HIT workout is the equivalent of 8 to 10 of those all-out sprints. In fact, Michael Johnson sometimes trained that way. But I guarantee you, he didn't do it often—especially if his sprints were in the 45-second range.

This is a fact of nature: The harder you train, the less you can stand. So as you train harder, you must do less.

Form

Form matters as much as intensity. Without proper form, the intensity of the exercise may be in vain and could even lead to injury. Although the form for each exercise I recommend is specific and will be described in its appropriate chapter, some generalizations apply to every exercise.

Minimum momentum. Inertia is the tendency of a weight or mass, if in motion, to keep moving in the same direction. The quantity of this motion is called momentum. Momentum adds to your performance in a weight-lifting or weight-throwing contest (such as a strongman competition, or a track and field event like the shot put), but it subtracts from your production if your goal is to exhaust your muscles as thoroughly as possible. The momentum itself can actually keep the resistance moving, which relieves the muscle of some of its tension.

Momentum, in other words, makes the exercise easier.

Your goal is to make it harder. You want to lift and lower the weight smoothly and slowly, with no jerks and sudden movements. Focus on the turn-arounds at the top and the bottom, and keep them especially deliberate and controlled. Doing so minimizes the momentum and makes the exercise harder.

Speed of movement. During the 1970s, I instructed trainees to take approximately 6 seconds to do a repetition on a Nautilus machine: 2 seconds on the positive and 4 seconds on the negative (2/4). Taking twice as long in the negative worked pretty well on machines that carried a lot of mechanical friction.

Today's machines are almost frictionless, which is why I now recommend that you do the positive and negative phases at the same speed. Depending on range of motion of the exercise, that speed can vary from 4 seconds (2/2) on a wrist curl to 14 seconds (7/7) on a pullover machine. An average of all the strength-training exercises creates a guideline of 4 seconds on the positive and 4 seconds on the negative (4/4).

On each of the recommended exercises in this book, your results will be faster, greater, and safer if you always remember the following:

• Move slowly

• Change direction smoothly

• Start and stop gradually

Range of movement. Try to work as much of the range of movement as is comfortably possible while understanding the following considerations.

1. In single-joint exercises (leg extensions, leg curls), pause briefly in the contracted position, but do not pause in the stretched position.

Build Strength, But Don't Demonstrate It

Abodybuilding workout is one thing. A competitive weight-lifting contest is a different matter. The best way to *build* strength has little in common with the best way to *demonstrate* strength. Yet many bodybuilders make the mistake of training as if they were in a weight-lifting meet, perhaps being more interested in impressing their peers than trying to build muscular size and strength.

Olympic lifters and powerlifters must practice maximum single-attempt lifts, both in training and in competition. But there's no reason for bodybuilders ever to attempt heavy singles. Although maximum muscular size cannot be produced without maximum muscular strength, it doesn't follow that building strength requires heavy single-attempt lifts. On the contrary, greater strength and size will result from the performance of repetitions within the 8-to-12 range.

Bodybuilders often hurt themselves during the first repetition of a set. You'd think it's because they failed to warm up properly. But in reality, they hurt themselves because they're strongest at that point in the set. They make the mistake of moving a weight from a dead stop to maximum speed. That requires a jerk, rather than smooth acceleration. The closer the lifter is to a maximum single-attempt lift, the greater the jerk. That's why single-attempt lifts are always the most dangerous type of movements.

For growth, you need to produce only *momentary* maximum contraction force. You can do that safely by first reducing your momentary ability. That means exhausting a muscle in some way so that the amount of force needed to produce that maximum contraction is less than it would've been had your muscles been fully rested when you attempted it.

You can do this by performing 3 or 4 repetitions immediately before a maximum movement. Or, even better, you can pre-exhaust the muscles by working them in an isolated fashion immediately before involving them in a heavier, multiple-joint movement.

2. In multiple-joint pulling exercises (lat pulldowns, rows), pause briefly in the contracted position, but do pause in the stretched position.

3. In multiple-joint pushing exercises (presses, squats), stop short of locking the knees and elbows in pressing movements, and do not pause in the extended or the flexed positions. The entire positive and negative movement is continuous.

Body posture. Correct posture on each exercise will help you achieve better and safer results. The general idea on most exercises is to keep your chest up and abdominals tight and to maintain a slight arch in your lower back. You want your head in what we call a neutral position, which means your neck isn't straining forward or backward.

When seated, keep both feet flat on the floor. If a machine has a seat belt, use it. When standing, your feet need to be at least shoulder width apart for stability, and you should keep a soft bend in your knees. Another way to say that: Avoid locking your knees on standing exercises.

Proper breathing. During any strength-training exercise, the rule is to concentrate on the muscles involved, not on your breathing. If you simply forget about how to breathe but remember to keep doing it, your breathing will take care of itself and supply your body with adequate oxygen—especially if your heart rate is high enough. There are points along the range of motion of every exercise where it's easier to breathe in or out. Your subconscious mind will identify these points and coordinate your breathing efficiently and naturally.

That said, it's also natural to hold your breath during the most intense repetitions, but you need to avoid that. Keeping your air passages closed while straining can cause something called the Valsalva effect, which may cause a headache or blackout.

In other words, don't hold your breath. Open your mouth, if necessary, and keep breathing.

Repetitions and Progression

I've always believed in doing 8 to 12 repetitions on most exercises. This repetition range guarantees that you fatigue the involved muscles without using such light weights that your body shifts toward its aerobic energy system. You want the work to stay in the anaerobic pathway, which means that a set should last no more than 120 seconds. The chemistry involved in the anaerobic pathway is best for gaining muscle size and strength.

Occasionally, I like to use higher repetitions (15 to 20) on lower-body muscles, and lower repetitions (5 to 8) on the upper body. But 8 to 12 repetitions per exercise has a long history of success.

Regardless of the repetition range, your goal is to make progress by getting stronger. Continuing to do what you can already do won't help you make improvements. The practical application: For each workout, you want to do more repetitions on each exercise than you did in the previous workout. When you get to 12, add more resistance.

You want to increase the weight in small increments—2 to 5 percent. In my experience, the smaller the increase, the better. You'll use better form and make steadier improvements.

Double progression, in which you strive to increase repetitions first, then resistance, has been the cornerstone of successful strength-training and bodybuilding programs for more than 100 years. You'll get the best results when that double progression is combined with the right intensity and good form.

Chapter 11

DURATION, FREQUENCY, AND ORDER

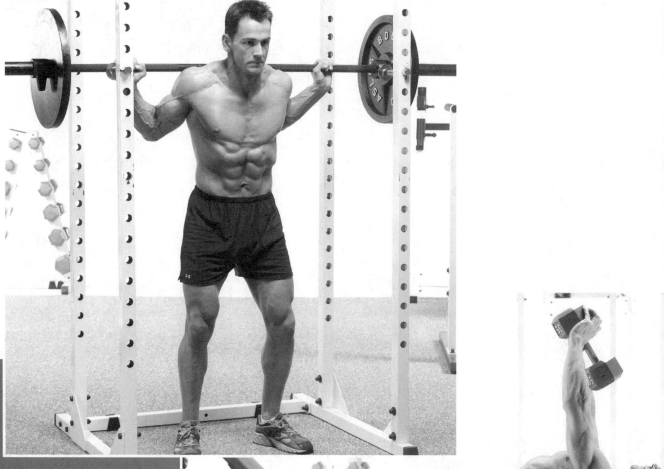

You'll achieve more-productive results from HIT if, each time you work out, you perform at least some exercise for both your lower and your upper body. In other words, whole-body routines are preferable to any type of split routine.

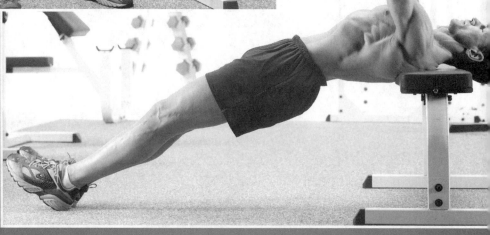

"GO TO THE gym, perform your workout properly, then get away from the gym and forget it until time for your next workout. Talking about bodybuilding, reading about bodybuilding, literally *living* bodybuilding will do nothing in the way of improving your results."

I've heard Arthur Jones deliver that message hundreds of times to motivated men who were working out multiple hours a day, five or six times a week. And during the 1 or 2 days a week that they weren't training, they were in the gym anyway, hanging around and soaking up the atmosphere.

That was the mindset when I was involved in competitive bodybuilding in the 1960s and 1970s, and it's really not so different today. In fact, as the story in "Enter the Tanny Booth" on page 88 shows, it goes back decades before my time. But if you want the best possible results, you need to master the intricacies of workout duration and frequency, and the order in which you perform your exercises.

Duration

You can look at your physique as seven sections—or body parts—that need to be trained: hips and thighs, calves, shoulders and neck, back, chest, arms, and waist. Each of these body parts should be exercised at least two times per week, unless you're at the advanced level. An advanced bodybuilder may reduce that to once a week. The total number of exercises per workout varies from a high of 12, if you're a beginner or intermediate trainee, to a low of 7, if you're an advanced bodybuilder.

Each exercise should be performed smoothly and slowly for one set of 8 to 12 repetitions, or from approximately 40 to 90 seconds, with 60 seconds

being the average time. No more than 60 seconds should elapse between exercises. Once you learn how to perform the exercises, you should need about 25 minutes to do the longest routine in this book. The shortest, with seven exercises, takes about 13 minutes.

If any of the routines in this book—from start to finish and with a warmup and a cooldown—take longer than 40 minutes to complete, then you're doing something wrong. Either you're not training hard enough or you're taking too much time between exercises. Once you learn a workout, you should be able to complete it in 25 minutes or less.

Remember, your goal is to train effectively and efficiently, and then get out of the gym.

Frequency

On a recent visit to Arthur Jones's home in Ocala, I asked him about optimum training frequency. Once again, he challenged me to think outside the box by bringing up his experience with lions.

"A large male lion will weigh around 500 pounds, and a large female will weigh 250 pounds. And what kind of exercise schedule does each follow?"

"I didn't know lions exercised," I said.

"Well, whether you call it work, or activity, or fighting, or chasing, or killing, they exercise. But there's a distinct difference between how the females exercise and how the males exercise.

"The females do the hunting. They stalk and kill game. Then they drag or carry the animals sometimes for miles to the dominant males. Of course, the females also take care of the young cubs when they're not hunting.

"The males, on the other hand, do only four

Enter the Tanny Booth

Vic Tanny had one of the first hard-core bodybuilding gyms on the West Coast. Despite its location in the basement of a building in Santa Monica, California, it was large and well-equipped. Tanny, who at one time owned a nationwide chain of gyms (they eventually became part of the Bally Total Fitness system), told me this story on one of his visits to the Nautilus headquarters in 1983.

"It was the summer after Steve Reeves had won the 1947 Mr. America. Steve, who lived near San Francisco, was in my gym training with George Eiferman, who was visiting from Philadelphia. Eiferman had entered the contest and had placed fifth, and he really wanted to win the next year."

When Eiferman asked Tanny's advice, Tanny couldn't resist messing with him. "I said, 'George, first you've got to move to California. Second, you've got to train every day and sometimes twice a day, 7 days a week. Third, my boy, you've got to spend a lot of time at the beach working on a tan.' I figured that George, whose skin was very white compared with Steve's, would realize I was pulling his leg. Having a dark tan wasn't an important factor in winning a physique contest back then."

Tanny got distracted with a phone call, Eiferman slipped out, and Tanny never got a chance to tell him the truth. Eiferman took a train back to Philadelphia but 2 months later showed up at the gym with all his belongings crammed into two duffel bags. He told Tanny he was ready to win the Mr. America.

"George had no place to stay, so I let him bed down in the gym for a while. That was a mistake, because George started training during the night as well as the day. After 6 weeks of that, I had to scout around and find him a rooming house down the street. But he was still training every day.

"His body was actually looking worse than when he arrived, so I called him into my office. This time I was serious. I told him, 'George, you're killing yourself with all that training. Stop!'" Tanny confessed that he'd been kidding about training every day and told Eiferman to get back to his whole-body training three times a week, which is what had made him a great bodybuilder in the first place.

Finally, he told him to spend more time at the beach, because doing so would keep Eiferman distracted and away from the gym.

"To his credit, he immediately got my drift and stopped training every day. Week by week, he started looking better and better. Six months later, at the Mr.

things. They fight, mate, eat, and sleep. The males attack each other violently for territorial and mating rights. The fighting is very intense but infrequent. Only the dominant male in each pride of lions mates with the females. The weaker males are killed, or they leave the territory."

"In other words," I said, "what you're saying is one of the reasons that a male lion is twice the size of a female has to do with the male working harder, briefer, and more infrequently than the female."

"Yes, and the female does a large amount of continuous-type activity. She certainly doesn't rest and sleep nearly as much as the male. The male probably sleeps 14 hours a day."

Jones's discussion about lions convinced me more than ever that three workouts per week—three whole-body workouts, that is—are much more productive for bodybuilding than any type of split or double-split routine. Your stimulated body needs approximately 48 hours or more between workouts for consistent recovery to occur. A

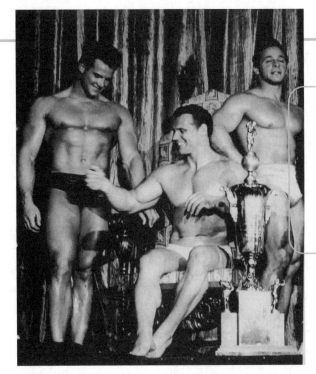

Vic Tanny held the 1949 Mr. USA contest in Los Angeles, and most of the top bodybuilders entered. John Grimek (seated) was the winner. Steve Reeves, standing on the left, was third, and George Eiferman, on the right, was fourth. Second place went to Clancy Ross.

America contest, it was neck and neck between George and Jack Delinger for the title.

"And you know what? George finally was declared the winner because a couple of the judges thought he had a better tan!"

Endnote: Recently, I told the above story to Bill Pearl, a former Mr. America and Mr. Universe, who was good friends with Tanny, Reeves, Eiferman, and Delinger. Pearl has had an ongoing feud, related to training duration and frequency, with Arthur Jones for more than 30 years. At the beginning of the account, when I was explaining Tanny's instructions (you must train every day and sometimes twice a day, 7 days a week), Pearl interrupted me, saying, "That's still good advice."

No, Bill, that's not good advice. But it certainly reinforces the concept that old bodybuilders don't change, they just pump away, repeating their mistakes again and again.

HIT offers a much more efficient way to bodybuilding success.

Monday-Wednesday-Friday workout schedule (or Tuesday-Thursday-Saturday) is an excellent starting place. Such a schedule has proved effective over and over again.

"Tell your readers one last thing," Jones said as I was leaving. "Tell them that if a three-times-per-week training schedule doesn't produce the results they're after, they should work out only twice a week." I thanked Jones, opened the front door, and said goodbye to the female who was preparing the kill for Jones's evening meal.

Going from Three to Two Times per Week

It's important to remember that as you get stronger, you must do less overall exercise to continue to get even stronger. The reason goes back to that thing called recovery ability. Your recovery ability does not increase in proportion to your ability to get stronger.

It should be obvious, then, that doing less overall exercise requires a reduction in either the frequency (times per week) or the duration (exer-

Short and Infrequent Workouts

Exercise should improve your strength and increase your overall ability in other physical activities. But too often, it does the opposite: It leaves you feeling constantly tired, with little energy for anything else. A persistent tired feeling should be a warning that something is wrong. Unfortunately, most lifters ignore this warning.

If you're untrained, you'll feel tired as a result of your first few workouts. But that feeling shouldn't last beyond the first week or so. If it does, you're overtraining. In short, your workouts are exceeding your recovery ability.

On the other hand, if you're an experienced bodybuilder, you should feel tired at the end of a workout, but you shouldn't remain tired. Within 20 minutes, you should feel as if you could go through your entire workout again (even though you should never try it). It takes very little high-intensity training to stimulate growth.

Never do more exercise when you can get better results from less.

---

cises per workout). There's also another way you can save some of your recovery ability: *Don't* go to momentary muscular failure during a workout. The idea is to use the same amount of resistance, but stop the set 2 repetitions short of an all-out effort. A not-to-failure (NTF) workout may actually facilitate recovery.

I find it helps to think of your workouts in 2-week segments, rather than looking at them as weeklong units. If you're training on a Monday-Wednesday-Friday schedule, you're working out six times in 2 weeks. The complete program, which I describe in detail in chapter 14, begins with 12 exercises, each performed to failure and repeated progressively six times in 2 weeks. After three 2-week segments, or 6 weeks, you cut back a bit on your training. The initial Wednesday workout is an NTF training session. You continue that way for 6 more weeks.

Then you drop the NTF workout, which leaves you training five times in 2 weeks. After 6 more weeks, one of your five workouts becomes NTF. At this point, it's taken you 18 weeks to reduce your HIT frequency from six times in 2 weeks to four times in 2 weeks, with one additional NTF workout.

The next step: Reduce the number of exercises in each workout from 12 to 10. You make another reduction with each new 6-week period, as you'll see in the table on page 132. Eventually, after 48 weeks, you're down to training three times in 2 weeks, with just 8 exercises per workout. By that time, you'll be smart enough and experienced enough to proceed to the advanced section.

Order

Many young guys get interested in strength training because they want to develop their pectorals and biceps. Thus, it's only natural that they begin most of their workouts with bench presses and curls—probably for many sets. Then, toward the end of their workouts, they might do a few leg exercises. Such a routine is a normal mistake but a mistake nonetheless.

The average bodybuilder isn't going to build much muscle mass on his pectorals and biceps unless he first builds considerable amounts around his hips, thighs, and back. It isn't possible to add significant muscular size in the small body parts un-

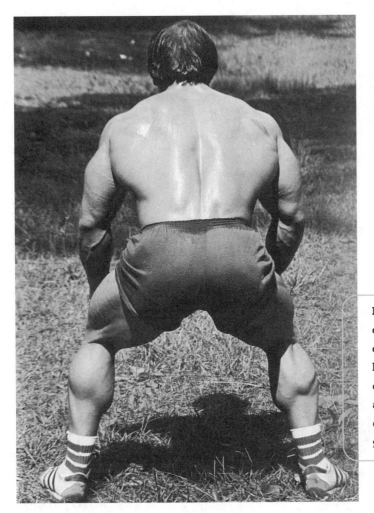

Bodybuilders, as well as other athletes, often neglect strengthening the backside of the body. The largest, strongest backside muscle is the gluteus maximus of the buttocks. Other important muscles are the trapezius, latissimus dorsi, erector spinae, hamstrings, and gastrocnemius.

less the big body parts are growing as well. In fact, your smaller body parts often progress in proportion to the increase in size of your larger body parts, even if you don't work the small areas.

That's why you should work the largest muscles first, when you're strongest and most motivated. Remember the workouts that Arthur Jones put Casey Viator through prior to the 1971 Mr. America? The workouts hit Viator's lower body for the first 10 minutes—and hit it hard. The payoff was evident; you can't do any better than first place in a major competition.

Remember this: If your energy and enthusiasm

are running low in any given workout, it's far better to skip the exercises for the smallest muscle groups, after expending whatever you had on the biggest muscles.

Ideally, you want to work your lower body before your upper body, your hips and thighs before your calves, your back before your shoulders and chest, and your upper arms before your forearms. Because your waist muscles stabilize your upper body in most exercises, work them last.

There are a few exceptions to the larger-to-smaller guideline. I'll discuss them in part IV, which focuses on specialized routines for specific goals.

Chapter 12

RECOVERY, LAYOFFS, SLEEP . . .
AND THE IMPORTANCE OF SAYING NO

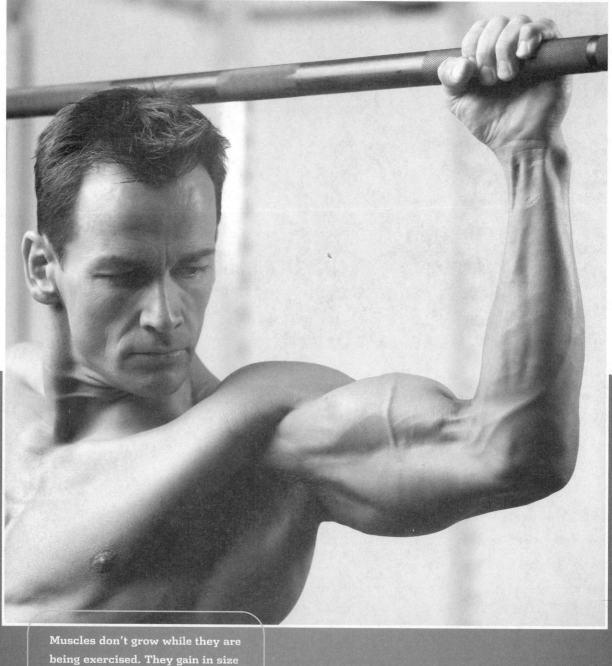

Muscles don't grow while they are being exercised. They gain in size during resting conditions.

IN THE SUMMER of 1971, Arthur Jones issued a challenge to the readers of *IronMan* magazine: "Build your arms as big as you can by any method except Nautilus equipment, and then come to De-Land, Florida, in muscular condition with the largest arms you can develop. Then, if you will simply follow instructions, I'll put a full one-half inch on the cold measurement of each of your upper arms—*from only one workout.*"

As extraordinary as this challenge was, it looks even bolder when you consider two things.

First, Jones's challenge was made to advanced bodybuilders. Many of these guys hadn't added any size to their arms in years, despite steady training. They would do almost anything to get an extra fraction of an inch on their biceps and triceps.

Second, Jones backed up his promise with this guarantee: "If you don't put half an inch of solid muscle on each of your upper arms, I'll pay your expenses to and from Florida."

So you'd assume that Jones had to reimburse the travel expenses of quite a few disappointed bodybuilders. But, in fact, only two guys out of more than 50 that accepted the challenge asked about refunds. And both of them later withdrew their requests.

What was Jones's secret? How was he able to induce so much muscular growth and do it so fast? The first part is what you already know—high-intensity training. The rest was what most lifters never think about: recovery from the workout, taking enough days off in between workouts, and getting enough sleep.

The Surefire Formula

Jones treated most of the 50 *IronMan* readers who accepted his challenge the exact same way. First, he'd meet the bodybuilder at the airport, the bus station, or a local restaurant. He'd measure the guy's arms almost immediately. Then, over a leisurely meal, they'd talk training, and Jones would explain his harder-but-briefer training philosophy.

After an hour of talk, Jones would check the bodybuilder into a resort or beachside hotel and instruct him to spend the next three nights and days sleeping, resting, and relaxing. Invariably, the guy would ask, "But what about my workout?"

Jones knew from his dinner conversation that the bodybuilder was overtrained—as most were then (and as most are now)—so it would be counterproductive to work him in that condition. What he desperately needed was the opposite of a workout—a layoff. Yes, he could enjoy the beach, the sun, and the fresh air. But Jones made the guy give his word that he wouldn't do exercise of any kind.

On the afternoon of the fourth day, Jones would meet the bodybuilder in the Quonset hut behind the high school in DeLand. The bodybuilder would be so crazed from not training—after working out almost every day, often twice a day, for years—that he couldn't wait to attack the iron.

Before the workout, Jones would measure the guy's arms again. As with most bodybuilders, his arms would already be $1/4$ inch larger. That's because, for the first time in years, the guy would be fully recovered from his last workout.

The workouts were usually 10 exercises—sometimes fewer but never more. Typically, there were 2

Recovery Ability: Essential for Normal (and Abnormal) Growth

During childhood and your teenage years, you achieve normal size and strength as part of the ordinary growth processes. You need little formal exercise to reach normal physical development. As a bodybuilder, however, you seek abnormal levels. Your objective is to build maximum levels of muscular size in the shortest time from the least effort. It only follows that you should be looking for the most productive method of exercise.

A healthy body will provide levels of size and strength according to its perception of what is needed for normal requirements, plus a bit more as a reserve for emergency use. As long as existing levels are adequate, as long as extreme demands are not made on the body, no additional size or strength will be provided. To produce growth, demands must be made in excess of normal. Only then will the body attempt to provide the size and strength required to meet these demands, if it can. Those last three words—"if it can"—are the most important.

The key, of course, is complete recovery. I define "recovery" as the chemical reactions necessary for your body to produce muscular growth. Optimum recovery ability depends on appropriate rest, adequate nutrition, and sufficient time.

Your body is a complex factory, constantly making hundreds of delicate changes that transform food and oxygen into the many chemicals needed by various parts of the system. But there's a limit to the chemical conversions that your recovery ability can make within a given time. If your requirements exceed that limit, your body will eventually be overworked to the point of collapse.

The recovery ability of your body provides normal growth. It also provides abnormal growth, if such abnormal growth is dictated and if the recovery ability is able to meet the requirements. It's not possible for you to exhaust your recovery ability while doing nothing to stimulate abnormal growth.

Obviously, then, to be productive, an exercise must stimulate abnormal growth as much as possible, while disturbing recovery ability as little as possible. Under this concept, an ideal exercise would be infinitely hard and infinitely brief. It would provide maximum stimulation while leaving your recovery ability in the best possible shape to meet the requirements for growth.

Rest well on your off days from training. Remember, the right amount of relaxation, sleep, and time are necessary for getting bigger and stronger.

---

exercises for the legs, 2 for the torso, and the rest devoted to the arms. Sometimes Jones skipped the legs.

Of course, the lifter did just one set of each exercise and always to complete failure. Jones often used negatives on the arm exercises. Most of the time, the guy had to be helped to a chair at the end of the workout just so he could sit down.

Jones would have another meal with the guy an hour after the workout, and this time his explanation of the high-intensity philosophy would be met with a more open mind. After another hour, it was back to the hotel for another night's sleep.

Finally, Jones would arrive early the next morning at the hotel and measure the guy's arms one final time. On each one I witnessed or heard about, the increase was at least $\frac{1}{2}$ inch from that first, fresh-off-the-plane measurement. A few gained $\frac{5}{8}$ inch or more. Only two guys came close to failing. They registered gains of $\frac{7}{16}$ inch. But after one more night's sleep, they were up another $\frac{1}{8}$ inch.

Most simply put: Jones's formula was based on the idea that training stimulates growth, but only full recovery permits that growth to actually occur.

Layoffs from Training

If 3 days without exercise adds ¼ inch to the average bodybuilder's arm, you probably wonder what would happen if you took a full week off. And that's a good question to ask.

I've learned, after working with hundreds of serious lifters, that a full week off from training works wonders. In fact, 9 days may be even better, and it's certainly a more natural break—after a Friday workout, you don't train again until Monday of the second week. Two weekends of rest and relaxation can do wonders for a bodybuilder's progress.

I think most guys do well with two 9-day layoffs a year, each following a solid 6 months of steady training. That gives you a 9-day vacation in the summer and a second one around the holidays. If you need to extend one or both of those breaks to 2 weeks, that shouldn't be a problem.

But you can get too much of a good layoff. Unless you're sick, injured, or otherwise unable to train, I wouldn't recommend any break longer than 30 days.

Finding Your Sleep Number

About 20 years ago, researchers found that sleep regulates brain function and body temperature and restores the immune system. More recently, they've reported that above-average amounts of sleep yield hormones that contribute to fat loss and muscle building.

The latest figures from the National Sleep Foundation show that the average adult in the United States gets 6 hours and 57 minutes of sleep per night during the work week, and 7 hours and 31 minutes on weekends. This isn't enough sleep, according to that organization, which recommends that adults get 8 hours of sleep every night.

What happens when you don't sleep enough? Lack of sleep for a few nights increases brain levels of cortisol, a potentially dangerous stress hormone, according to Eve Van Cauter, Ph.D., a University of Chicago sleep researcher. High cortisol levels weaken your immune system and contribute to a number of problems—depression, irritability, low energy, muscle loss, and fat storage.

Let's say you've given HIT a fair trial, but after several weeks you still don't see the type of gains in size and strength you had expected. I'd immediately suspect that you need more sleep each night.

To get that sleep, you have to learn to say no to a lot of habits and behaviors, even to the point of setting limits for friends and loved ones. No late-night TV. No all-nighters with your drinking buddies. No middle-of-the-night phone calls from family or friends.

Here are some guidelines.

• Get 10 hours of sleep each night if you are a teenager, 9 hours if you're an adult.

• When possible, take a 15-minute nap in the middle of the afternoon (even better: schedule it).

Now, combine that extra sleep with a 9-day break from training every 6 months, and your recovery ability will finally be strong enough to allow your body to grow.

Chapter 13

THE NOT-SO-SECRET EXERCISES

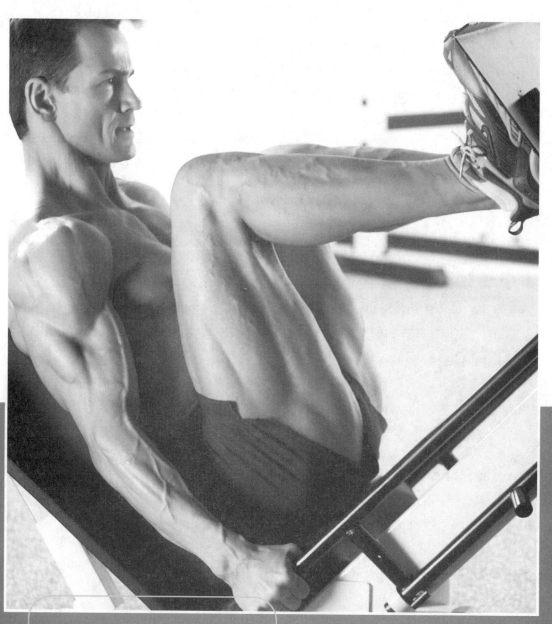

The leg press is a multiple-joint exercise because it requires movement around the hips, knees, and ankles.

COUNT UP ALL the exercises you can do with barbells and dumbbells, add in all the moves you can do with the machines you find in commercial gyms, and you end up with hundreds of exercises to choose from.

Some, however, are more productive than others. My experience as a lifter, trainer, and researcher—and we're talking about more than 40 years in the gym—tells me that the best exercises are the ones that best match the muscles' major functions. Once I look at what a muscle is designed to do, and which exercises best mimic those functions, I can eliminate most of the exercises out there. That leaves me with fewer than two dozen basic, tried-and-true exercises and spares me from having to think about the ones that overlap the key moves, are peripheral to a muscle's function, or are just plain risky.

In other words, there are no secret exercises that'll put an inch on your arms. I can and will, however, show you plenty of innovative ways to use those not-so-secret exercises. I'll present classic workouts as well as new ones in later chapters.

For now, let's look at what are the best exercises and how to combine them into basic routines.

Single- and Multiple-Joint Movements

The basic HIT exercises can be grouped under two headings: single-joint and multiple-joint movements. Single-joint movements, as you certainly guessed, involve only one joint. A lateral raise with dumbbells qualifies, since only the shoulder joints move. The overhead press with a barbell is a good example of a multiple-joint move, because the shoulders, wrists, and elbows are involved.

Both types of exercises are important for your goal of building muscle but for different reasons: A single-joint movement does a much better job of isolating a targeted muscle, such as the deltoids in the case of the lateral raise. A multiple-joint exercise involves some work for many muscles, although it doesn't work any muscle group thoroughly. The overhead press stresses your triceps, deltoids, and trapezius, but doesn't take any of those muscles through a long range of movement. For that, you'd need a good extension exercise for the triceps, a lateral raise for the deltoids, and a shoulder shrug for the traps.

But that doesn't make the overhead press an inferior exercise. It brings more total muscle mass into action than any single-joint exercise. That means you can use a much heavier resistance and induce better overall muscle growth.

So you have one type of exercise for overall mass and another type for working specific muscles through longer ranges of motion, thus taxing them more thoroughly. Put them together in the right way, and you have the perfect workout.

Best Single-Joint Exercises

Leg-extension machine

Leg-curl machine

Standing-calf-raise machine

Lateral raise with dumbbells

Straight-arm pullover with one dumbbell

Bent-arm fly with dumbbells

Biceps curl with barbell

Triceps extension with one dumbbell

Wrist curl with barbell

Trunk curl on floor

Best Multiple-Joint Exercises

Squat with barbell

Stiff-legged deadlift with barbell

Leg-press machine

Bent-over row with barbell

Overhead press with barbell

Bench press with barbell

Negative chinup

Negative dip

Next-Best Exercises

Seated-calf-raise machine

Bent-arm pullover with barbell

Pulldown on lat machine

Incline bench press with barbell

Front raise with dumbbells

Bent-over raise with dumbbells

Shoulder shrug with barbell (or dumbbells)

Reverse curl with barbell

Pushdown on lat machine

Reverse wrist curl with barbell

Prone back raise on bench

Side bend with dumbbell

Reverse trunk curl on floor

Exercises to Avoid

The following exercises are unsafe and should not be practiced.

Power clean with barbell

Clean and jerk with barbell

Power snatch with barbell

Snatch with barbell

Lunge with dumbbells

Jump squat with dumbbells

Front squat with barbell

Neck bridge with barbell

The power clean, clean and jerk, power snatch, and snatch are popular among Olympic weight lifters and necessary because these maximum lifts are part of their competition. However, the explosive nature of these lifts places tremendous forces on the involved muscles, connective tissues, and joints. Furthermore, these exercises all involve too much momentum to be effective muscle builders. Some football coaches recommend that their players do power cleans. They are of little value to a football player. Stay clear of these exercises or any other exercise that is done explosively.

The lunge with dumbbells or a barbell is another dangerous movement. Too much momentum is involved in stepping forward and backward with a heavy weight. Besides, the squat with a barbell is much safer and more productive.

The jump squat with dumbbells is another unsafe exercise. Jumping by its very nature is explosive. Don't do it.

The front squat with a barbell, because of the placement of the bar across your clavicles, is uncomfortable and restraining. The squat with a barbell, again, is more productive.

The neck bridge with a barbell across the chest is a favorite of many wrestlers. It, however, places too much compression force on the cervical spine. Specifically designed neck machines by Nautilus, Hammer, and MedX are better bets for building neck muscles.

Now that you have a comprehensive list of exercises, ranging from the best to the worst, let's take a closer look at the best and next-best HIT-recommended exercises.

Best Single-Joint Exercises

LEG-EXTENSION MACHINE
Muscles Worked: Quadriceps

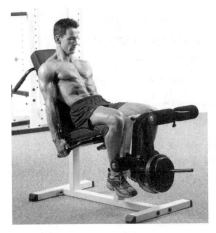

Start:

- Sit in the machine and place your feet and ankles behind the bottom roller pad.

- Align your knees with the axis of rotation of the movement arm.

- Lap the belt across your hips securely, if one is provided, to keep your buttocks from rising.

- Lean back and stabilize your upper body by grasping the handles or the sides of the machine.

Execution:

- Straighten your legs smoothly.

- Ease into the fully contracted top position.

- Pause briefly.

- Lower the weight slowly.

- Repeat for maximum repetitions.

HIT TIPS:

- Relax your feet during the lifting and lowering. Do not point your toes or flex them.

- Keep your neck and face relaxed, especially on the last repetitions.

- Do not move your head forward or side to side.

- Emphasize your breathing on your final repetition. Do not hold your breath.

- Practice smooth turnarounds at both ends of the exercise.

Best Single-Joint Exercises

LEG-CURL MACHINE
Muscles Worked: Hamstrings

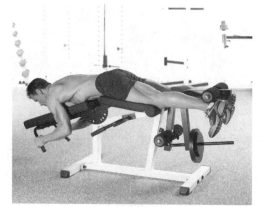

Start:

- Lie facedown on the machine with your knees on the pad edge closest to the movement arm.

- Hook your heels and ankles under the roller pad.

- Make certain your knees are in line with the axis of rotation of the movement arm.

- Grasp the handles provided on the edges of the machine bench to steady your upper body.

HIT TIPS:

- Keep your feet relaxed during the first half of each repetition. As you progress into the contracted position, move your toes toward your knees. This flexing of the ankle stretches your calves and allows for a greater range of motion from the hamstrings.

- Hook your hands on the handles underneath to keep your knees from sliding off the axis of rotation of the movement arm.

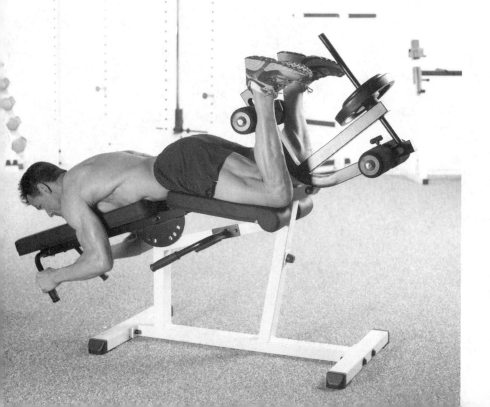

Execution:

- Curl your heels smoothly and try to touch the roller pad to your buttocks. Near the fully contracted position, you must lift your buttocks off the pad and arch your back slightly. Do not try to keep your hips down.

- Pause briefly in the top position.

- Ease out of the top position and lower the movement arm slowly.

- Repeat for maximum repetitions.

Best Single-Joint Exercises

STANDING-CALF-RAISE MACHINE

Muscles Worked: Gastrocnemius (the large, diamond-shaped muscle on the back of your calves) and soleus (the flat muscle that lies between the gastroc and the lower-leg bones)

Start:

- Face the machine and bend your knees enough so that you can position your shoulders beneath the yoke.

- Stand and place your feet shoulder width apart on the toe block or step, with only your toes and the balls of your feet in contact with the block.

- Straighten your knees and keep them locked throughout the exercise.

- Sag your heels as far below the level of your toes as comfortably possible.

- Keep your feet pointed straight ahead.

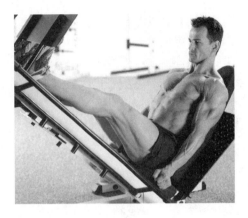

Execution:

- Raise your heels smoothly and try to stand on your tiptoes.

- Do not bend your knees.

- Pause briefly in the highest position.

- Lower slowly to the bottom and stretch.

- Repeat for maximum repetitions.

If a standing-calf-raise machine is unavailable, performing the exercise on a leg-press machine, as shown, is a reasonable substitute.

HIT TIPS:

- Do not believe that turning your toes in on the calf raise works more of the lateral (outside) head of the gastrocnemius, or turning your toes out involves more of the medial (inside) head. The origin and insertion points of the gastrocnemius are not altered by foot placement.

- Sustain a slow speed of movement, especially since the calf raise entails such a short range.

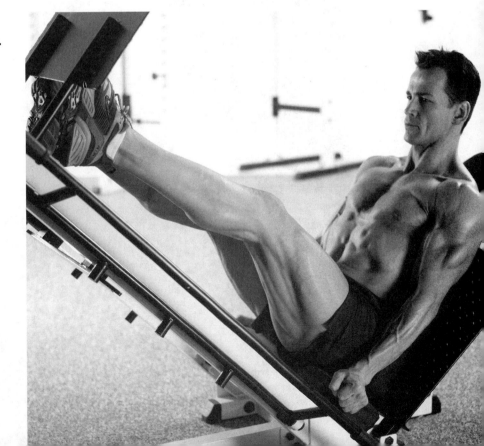

LATERAL RAISE WITH DUMBBELLS

Muscles Worked: Middle deltoids

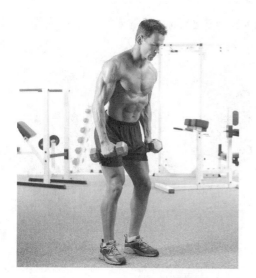

Start:

- Grasp a dumbbell in each hand and stand.

- Lean forward at the waist approximately 20 degrees from vertical. Stay in this leaning-forward position throughout the movement.

- Lock your elbows and wrists and keep them almost locked throughout the exercise. All the action should occur around your shoulder joints.

HIT TIPS:

- Resist the temptation to start the movement with a jerk or a roll.

- Initiate the movement with your deltoids, not your head and arms.

Execution:

- Raise your arms sideways.

- Pause briefly when the dumbbells are slightly above the horizontal. Make sure your palms are facing down and your elbows are almost straight.

- Lower the dumbbells slowly to your sides.

- Repeat for maximum repetitions.

STRAIGHT-ARM PULLOVER WITH ONE DUMBBELL

Muscles Worked: Latissimus dorsi

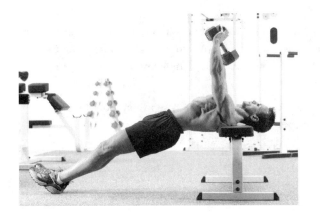

Start:

- Lie crossways on a bench with your shoulders in contact with the bench and your head and lower body relaxed and off the bench.

- Hold a dumbbell at one end with both hands and position it over your chest with your arms straight.

HIT TIPS:

- Emphasize the stretching that occurs in the bottom position.

- Practice taking deep breaths at the start.

Execution:

- Take a deep breath and lower the dumbbell slowly behind your head.

- Stretch your lats and rib cage gradually.

- Raise the dumbbell smoothly to the over-chest position.

- Repeat for maximum repetitions.

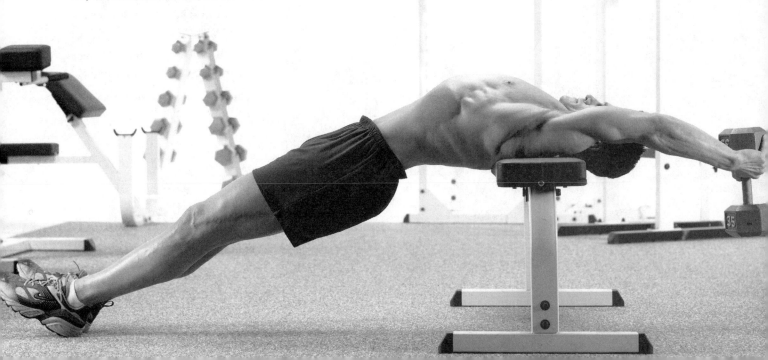

Best Single-Joint Exercises

BENT-ARM FLY WITH DUMBBELLS
Muscles Worked: Pectoralis major

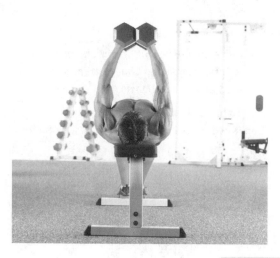

Start:

- Grasp two dumbbells, lie back on a flat exercise bench, and extend your arms upward from your shoulders. Your palms should be facing each other while you are holding the dumbbells.

- Bend your elbows slightly and keep them bent throughout the movement.

HIT TIPS:

- Keep your hands, elbows, and shoulders—when viewed from the side—in line with one another. This directs most of the emphasis to your chest muscles.

- Be careful about going too low or stretching too much in the bottom position.

Execution:

- Lower the dumbbells slowly out to the sides in semicircular arcs as low as comfortably possible.

- Return the dumbbells smoothly along the same arcs to the top position.

- Repeat for maximum repetitions.

Best Single-Joint Exercises

BICEPS CURL WITH BARBELL
Muscles Worked: Biceps

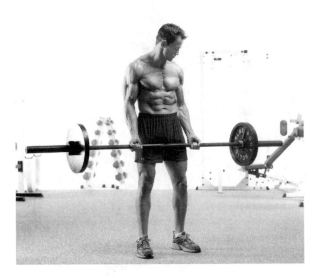

Start:

- Take a shoulder-width underhand grip on a barbell and stand.

- Anchor your elbows firmly against the sides of your waist and keep them there throughout the exercise.

- Lean forward slightly and look at your hands.

HIT TIPS:

- Maximize your biceps stimulation by minimizing your body sway.

- Do not lean forward excessively or lean backward. Do not move your head.

- Concentrate on your breathing and keep the repetitions strict.

Execution:

- Curl the barbell smoothly.

- Pause in the top position, but do not move your elbows forward. Keep your hands in front of your elbows.

- Lower the bar slowly. Again, keep your elbows stable against your sides.

- Repeat for maximum repetitions.

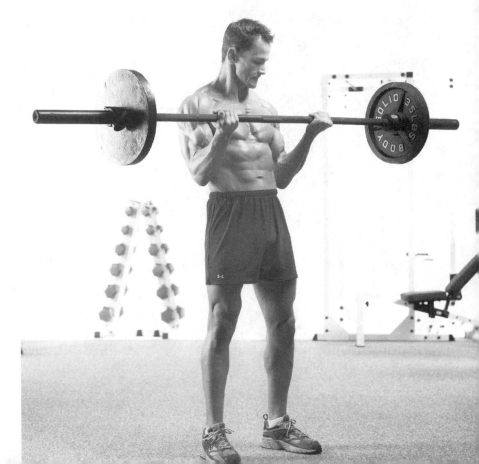

Best Single-Joint Exercises

TRICEPS EXTENSION WITH ONE DUMBBELL
Muscles Worked: Triceps

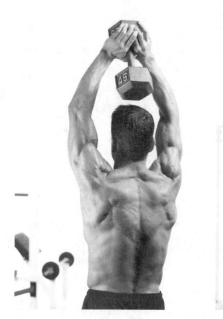

Start:

• Hold a dumbbell at one end with both hands.

• Press the dumbbell overhead.

• Pull your elbows in tight and keep them close to your ears throughout the exercise.

HIT TIPS:

• Be alert in the bottom position, as the triceps is stretched across two joints. Thus, it is vulnerable to strains. Move in and out of the bottom position gradually with no jerks.

• Keep your face and neck relaxed.

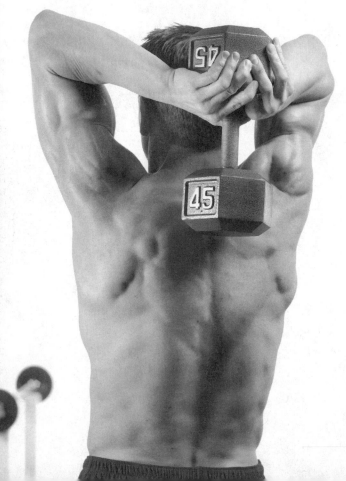

Execution:

• Bend your elbows and lower the dumbbell slowly behind your neck. Don't move your elbows. Only your forearms and hands should move.

• Press the dumbbell smoothly back to the extended position.

• Repeat for maximum repetitions.

WRIST CURL WITH BARBELL

Muscles Worked: Forearm flexors

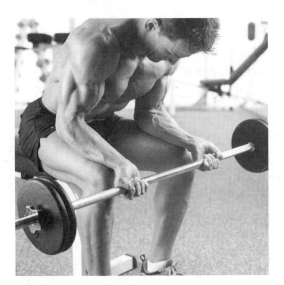

Start:

- Grasp a barbell with a palms-up grip.

- Sit down and rest your forearms on your thighs and the backs of your hands against your knees.

- Lean forward until the angle between your upper arms and forearms is 90 degrees. This position allows you to isolate your forearms better.

HIT TIPS:

- Remain in the bent-over position for all repetitions.

- Keep the movement deliberate and focused.

Execution:

- Curl your hands smoothly and contract your forearm muscles.

- Pause briefly.

- Lower the barbell slowly.

- Repeat for maximum repetitions.

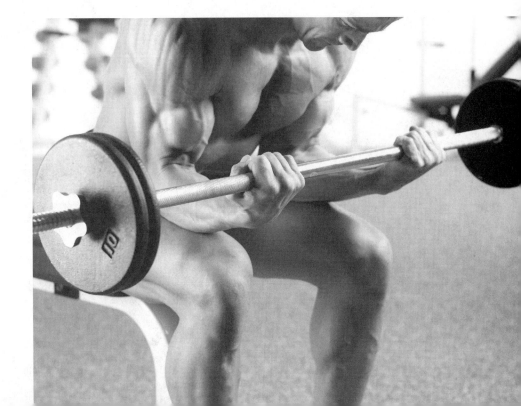

Best Single-Joint Exercises

TRUNK CURL ON FLOOR
Muscles Worked: Rectus abdominis and external obliques

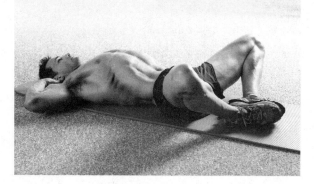

Start:

- Lie faceup on the floor with your hands cupped over your ears and your elbows back.

- Keep your head stable.

- Bring your heels up close to your buttocks and spread your knees.

- Do not anchor your feet under anything, and don't have a partner hold your knees down. Anchoring your feet brings into action your hip flexors.

HIT TIPS:

- Relax your neck and face. Do not move your head forward excessively.

- Execute the movement smoothly, without jerking your head and shoulders up off the floor.

- Hold a barbell plate across your upper chest to make the exercise harder.

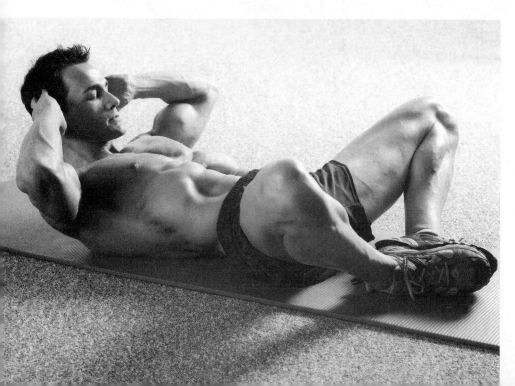

Execution:

- Tighten your abdominals initially.

- Curl your shoulders toward your hips. Your head and upper back will lift slightly as you contract, while your lower back flattens and presses into the floor. You will be able to move only one-fourth of the way up.

- Pause in the highest position.

- Lower your upper back, shoulders, and head slowly to the floor.

- Repeat for maximum repetitions.

Best Multiple-Joint Exercises

SQUAT WITH BARBELL

Muscles Worked: Buttocks, hamstrings, quadriceps, and lower back

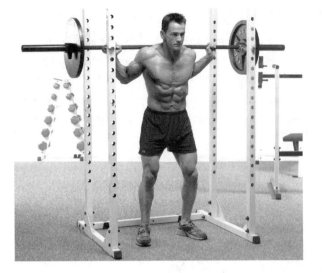

Start:

- Place a barbell on a squat rack and load it with an appropriate amount of weight.

- Position the bar behind your neck across your trapezius muscles, and hold the bar in place with your hands. If the bar cuts into your skin, pad it lightly by wrapping a towel around the knurl.

- Straighten your legs to lift the bar off the rack and move back one step.

- Place your feet shoulder width apart, toes angled slightly outward. Keep your upper-body muscles rigid and your torso upright during this exercise. It also helps if you focus on a spot on the wall at eye level as you do the movement.

HIT TIPS:

- Do not allow your torso to bend forward as you rise out of the bottom position.

- Use spotters in this exercise.

Execution:

- Bend your hips and knees and smoothly descend to a position whereby your hamstrings firmly come in contact with your calves. Without bouncing or stopping in the bottom position, slowly make the turnaround from negative to positive.

- Lift the barbell back to the top position.

- Repeat for maximum repetitions.

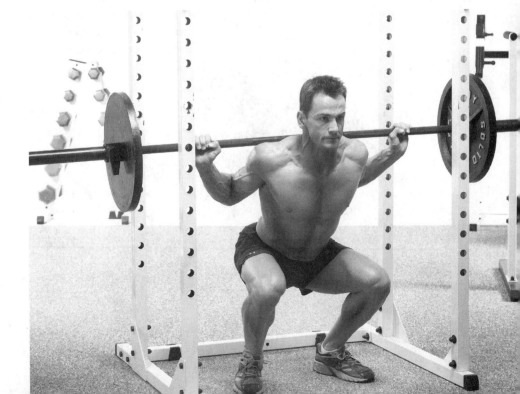

Best Multiple-Joint Exercises

STIFF-LEGGED DEADLIFT WITH BARBELL
Muscles Worked: Lower back, buttocks, and hamstrings

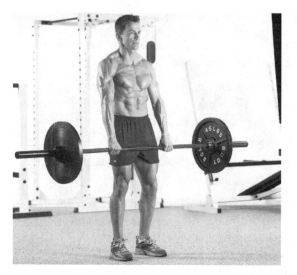

Start:

- Even though this exercise is called a stiff-legged deadlift, it should be performed with a slight bend in your knees. This protects the vertebrae of your lower back.

- Stand over a barbell, bend your hips and knees, and grasp the bar with an overhand grip and your hands shoulder width apart.

- Extend your hips and knees and lift the barbell smoothly to a standing position.

Execution:

- Lower the barbell smoothly down your thighs and shins, while keeping a slight bend in your knees.

- Touch the floor lightly with the barbell, but do not come to a stop.

- Lift the barbell slowly up your shins and thighs to the standing position.

- Repeat for 8 to 12 repetitions. *Note:* Ease into the stiff-legged deadlift, especially if you have any problem or tenderness in your lower back. For the first several weeks, use a light resistance and do not go to momentary muscular failure.

HIT TIPS:

- Be careful about using an alternating grip (one hand under and one hand over). Doing so places unequal stress on the arms.

- Keep the movement smooth and avoid bouncing the barbell off the floor.

Best Multiple-Joint Exercises

LEG-PRESS MACHINE

Muscles Worked: Buttocks, quadriceps, and hamstrings

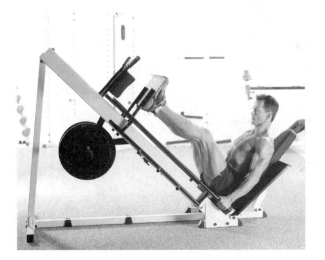

Start:

- Sit in the machine with your back against the angled pad and your buttocks on the seat bottom.

- Place your feet on the moving platform with your heels about shoulder width apart and your toes pointed slightly outward.

- Straighten your legs and release the stop bars of the machine (be sure to lock these stop bars at the end of your set to secure the platform).

- Grasp the handles beside the seat or the edge of the seat during the movement.

Execution:

- Lower the weight slowly by bending your hips and knees.

- Bring your knees to the sides of your chest and smoothly make the turnaround from negative (lowering) to positive (lifting).

- Press the weight smoothly, but do not lock your knees. Keep a bend of 15 degrees in your knees.

- Repeat for maximum repetitions.

HIT TIPS:

- Practice smooth turnarounds at both the top and the bottom.

- Do not slam into the platform or bounce and bang the resistance at either end of the exercise.

- Focus on relaxing your face and neck.

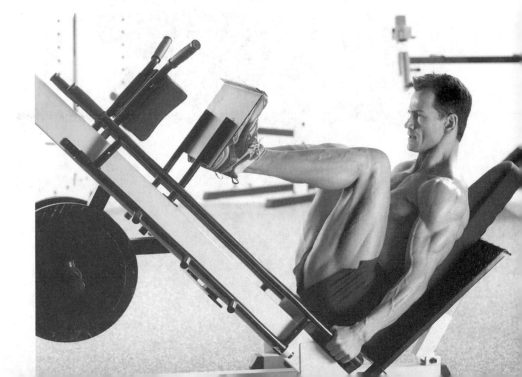

Best Multiple-Joint Exercises

BENT-OVER ROW WITH BARBELL

Muscles Worked: Latissimus dorsi and biceps

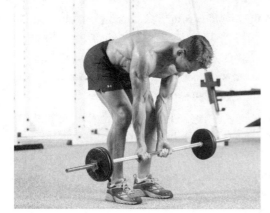

Start:

• Place your feet close together under a barbell.

• Bend over and grasp the barbell with an underhand grip. Your hands should be approximately 4 inches apart. Your torso should remain parallel to the floor.

• Keep a slight bend in your knees to reduce the stress on your lower back.

HIT TIPS:

• Emphasize your latissimus dorsi more by rowing with an underhand grip, which places your biceps in a stronger position.

• Pause in the top position and try to pinch your shoulder blades together.

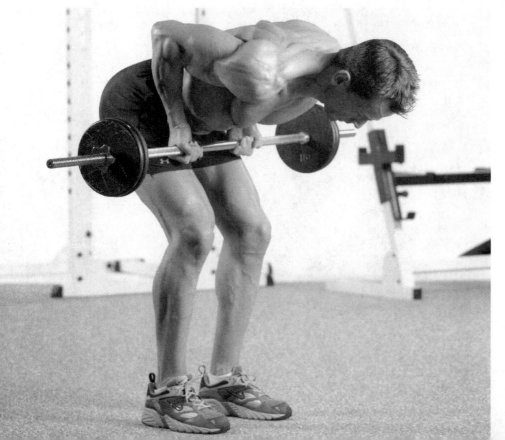

Execution:

• Pull the barbell up your thighs and touch your waist.

• Pause.

• Lower slowly to the bottom and stretch.

• Repeat for maximum repetitions.

Best Multiple-Joint Exercises

OVERHEAD PRESS WITH BARBELL

Muscles Worked: Deltoids, trapezius, and triceps

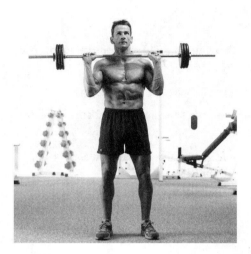

Start:

- Stand and place a barbell in front of your shoulders with your hands slightly wider than your shoulders.

- Keep your feet shoulder width apart.

HIT TIPS:

- Do not bounce the barbell off your shoulders at the bottom.

- Emphasize the bottom turnaround by keeping the movement steady.

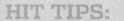

Execution:

- Press the barbell overhead smoothly.

- Do not lock your elbows. Keep a slight bend in them at the top.

- Lower the weight slowly to your shoulders.

- Repeat for maximum repetitions.

Best Multiple-Joint Exercises

BENCH PRESS WITH BARBELL

Muscles Worked: Pectorals, deltoids, and triceps

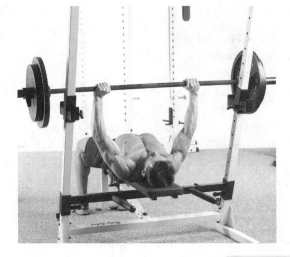

Start:

- Set up a barbell with an appropriate load on the supports of a flat bench.

- Lie on your back on the bench.

- Grasp the barbell with your hands positioned slightly wider than your shoulders.

- Straighten your arms to bring the barbell to a supported position directly above your shoulders.

HIT TIPS:

- Avoid using a wide grip on the bench press. Since the function of your pectoral muscles is to move your upper arms across your torso, spacing your hands wider than your shoulders actually shortens your range of movement. Rather than working more of your chest muscles, you're working less of them.

- Use a spotter on this exercise.

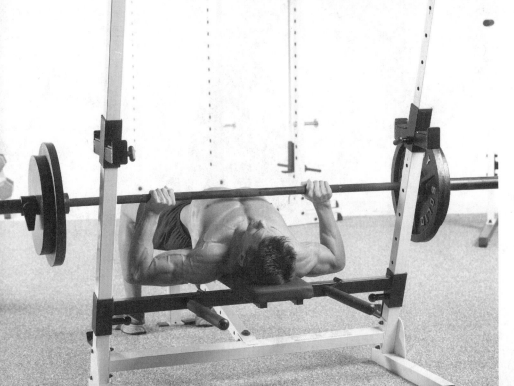

Execution:

- Lower the barbell slowly to your chest.

- Touch your chest, but do not rest.

- Press the barbell smoothly until your arms are almost straight. Keep a slight bend in your elbows in the top position.

- Repeat for maximum repetitions.

NEGATIVE CHINUP

Muscles Worked: Biceps and latissimus dorsi

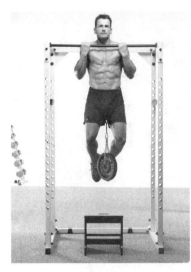

Start:

- Use a sturdy chair or bench for assistance. The idea is to do the positive work with your legs and the negative work with your upper body.

- Place the chair or bench directly under a chinning bar. Slip into a padded weight belt and attach an appropriate weight to the chain.

- Climb into the top position with your chin over the bar. Hold on to the bar with an underhand grip and space your hands shoulder width apart.

Execution:

- Remove your feet from the chair or bench.

- Lower your body very slowly in 8 to 10 seconds.

- Make sure you come all the way down to a dead hang.

- Climb back quickly into the top position with your chin over the bar.

- Repeat the slow lowering for maximum repetitions.

HIT TIPS:

- During your first several negative repetitions, take 10 seconds to lower your body. If you had to, you could stop the downward movement—but don't. Continue to lower in 10 seconds.

- After 5 or 6 repetitions, if the weight is selected correctly, you should be able to control the downward movement but *not* stop it.

- When you can no longer control your negative repetition, stop. In other words, stop when the entire lowering portion is completed in 2 or 3 seconds, in spite of your best efforts to reduce the speed.

- When you can do 12 repetitions in good form, add more weight around your waist.

- Your strength will increase rapidly on the negative chinup. Soon you'll be able to hang additional weight around your waist.

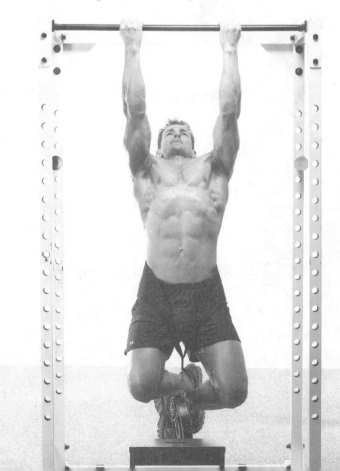

Best Multiple-Joint Exercises

NEGATIVE DIP

Muscles Worked: Triceps, deltoids, and pectorals

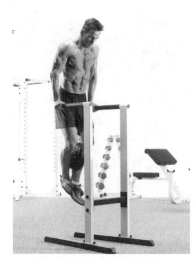

Start:

- Place a sturdy chair or bench between the parallel bars. Or use the built-in step or horizontal bar that some machines provide. Most trainees will require extra resistance added to their body weight with a waist belt.

- Climb into the top position and straighten your arms.

- Remove your feet from the chair and stabilize your body.

Execution:

- Bend your arms and lower your body slowly, taking 10 seconds.

- Feel the stretch in the bottom position (which shouldn't be painful, especially to your shoulders).

- Climb back into the starting position and straighten your arms.

- Repeat the slow lowering for maximum repetitions.

HIT TIPS:

- Keep the time between negative repetitions as brief as possible. Quickly climb back into the top position.

- Do not take longer than 3 seconds on the climb. In fact, 2 seconds is even better. Taking a longer time between negative repetitions allows your involved muscles a chance to recover partially.

Next-Best Exercises

SEATED-CALF-RAISE MACHINE
Muscles Worked: Soleus

Start:

• Sit in the machine with the padded movement arm resting on your lower thighs and the balls of your feet on the raised step.

• Adjust the machine until your knees are bent to approximately 90 degrees.

Execution:

• Lift your heels smoothly and try to extend on your big toes.

• Pause.

• Lower slowly to the bottom and stretch.

• Repeat for maximum repetitions.

HIT TIPS:

• Concentrate on moving slowly and going full range.

• Keep your face and neck relaxed.

10 Simple Rules

All the HIT concepts that I've presented in previous chapters can be boiled down to 10 simple rules. Implementation of these rules is difficult, but the rules themselves are straightforward.

• Do each repetition slowly and smoothly. Avoid fast and jerky movements.

• Perform 8 to 12 repetitions per set, which should take from 60 to 90 seconds. After the target repetition is reached, increase the resistance by 2 to 5 percent at your next workout.

• Continue each repetition until momentary muscular failure for maximum intensity.

• Limit a routine to 12 exercises, or fewer, per workout.

• Train for 3 nonconsecutive days, or less, per week.

• Work your body's largest muscles first and the smallest muscles last.

• Select exercises that involve both single-joint and multiple-joint movements.

• Initiate specialized routines for only 2 consecutive weeks. Wait for 3 months before you specialize again on the same body part.

• Optimize your recovery ability by training less as you get stronger.

• Take a 9-day layoff after each 6 months of steady training.

BENT-ARM PULLOVER WITH BARBELL
Muscles Worked: Latissimus dorsi and triceps

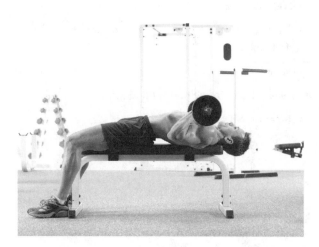

Start:

- Lie faceup on a high, narrow bench with your head barely off the edge.

- Anchor your feet securely underneath.

- Have a spotter hand you a heavy barbell. Your hands should be spaced 12 inches apart. The barbell should be resting on your chest.

HIT TIPS:

- Practice with a medium amount of resistance before you go heavy.

- Have your spotter hand you the barbell at the start and take it from you at the finish.

Execution:

- Move the barbell over your face and head and lower it smoothly until you touch the floor, or get as close to it as possible.

- Don't straighten your arms. Keep them bent.

- Stretch in the bottom position.

- Pull the barbell over your face to your chest.

- Repeat the lowering and lifting for maximum repetitions.

Next-Best Exercises

PULLDOWN ON LAT MACHINE

Muscles Worked: Biceps and latissimus dorsi

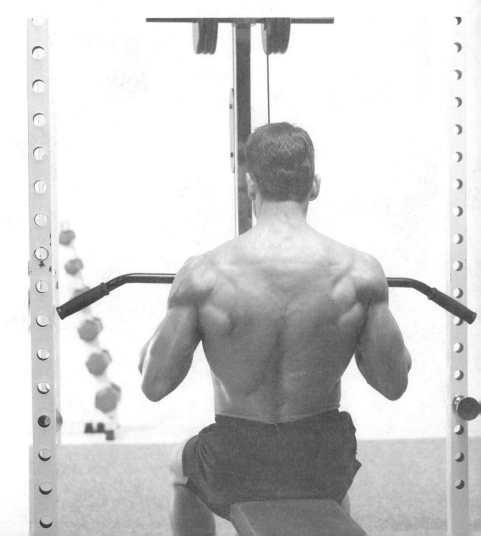

Start:

- Use a parallel-grip bar, if possible. If not, use an underhand grip.

- Stabilize yourself under the lat machine and grasp the bar.

HIT TIPS:

- Keep your torso erect during each repetition.

- Minimize your body sway.

Execution:

- Pull the bar smoothly behind your neck, with a parallel grip, or to your chest, with an underhand grip (as shown).

- Pause.

- Return slowly to the stretched position.

- Repeat for maximum repetitions.

INCLINE BENCH PRESS WITH BARBELL

Muscles Worked: Triceps, deltoids, and pectorals

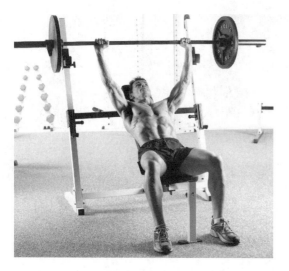

Start:

- Use a 45-degree incline bench with support racks, if possible, for this exercise.

- Position your hands on the bar slightly wider than your shoulders.

- Lift the barbell over your upper chest.

HIT TIPS:

- Avoid arching your back excessively.

- Have a spotter to assist you if necessary.

Execution:

- Lower the barbell slowly while keeping your elbows wide.

- Touch your upper chest and then press the bar back until your arms are almost straight.

- Repeat for maximum repetitions.

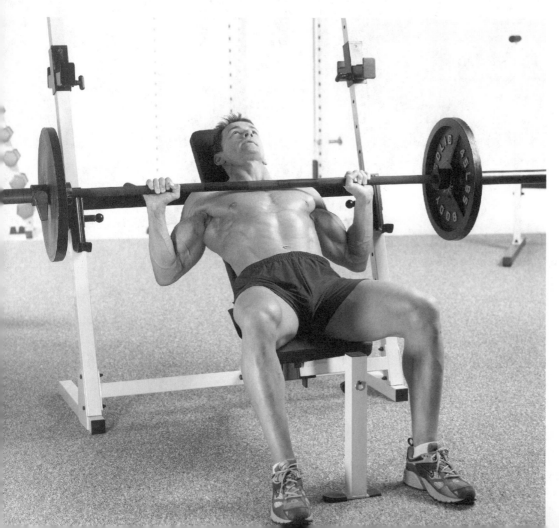

Next-Best Exercises

FRONT RAISE WITH DUMBBELLS

Muscles Worked: Anterior deltoids

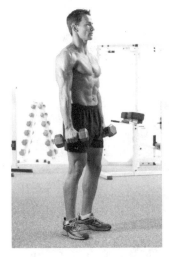

Start:

• Grasp a dumbbell in each hand and stand.

• Turn the dumbbells so that your thumbs are forward.

• Keep a slight bend in your elbows throughout the movement.

HIT TIPS:

• Avoid leaning forward and backward during the exercise.

• Keep your form strict.

Execution:

• Raise your arms forward and up until they're slightly above shoulder level.

• Pause. Keep your thumbs up.

• Lower slowly with control.

• Repeat for maximum repetitions.

Next-Best Exercises

BENT-OVER RAISE WITH DUMBBELLS
Muscles Worked: Posterior deltoids

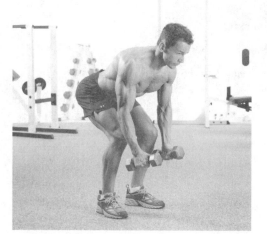

Start:

• Grasp a light dumbbell in each hand.

• Lean forward until your torso is parallel to the floor.

• Allow your arms to hang with a slight bend in your elbows, and keep a slight bend in your knees.

HIT TIPS:

• Keep the movement slow and deliberate.

• Do not move your head and upper back. Keep them stable.

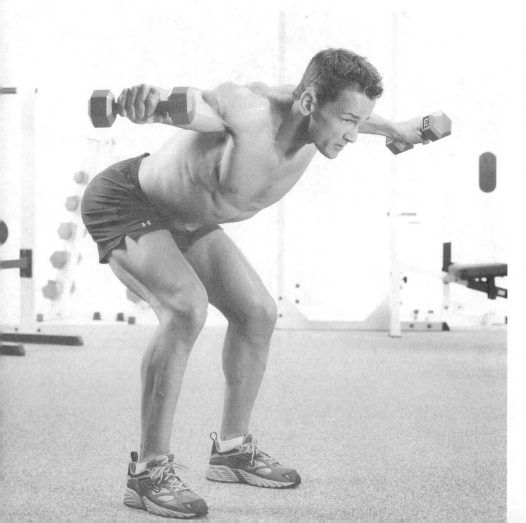

Execution:

• Raise the dumbbells smoothly to the sides.

• Pause when the dumbbells are level with your shoulders.

• Lower slowly to the hanging position.

• Repeat for maximum repetitions.

SHOULDER SHRUG WITH BARBELL

Muscles Worked: Trapezius

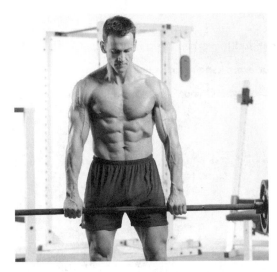

Start:

- Take an overhand grip on a barbell and stand erect. Your hands should be slightly wider apart than your shoulders, and the bar should be touching your thighs.

- Sag your shoulders forward and downward as far as comfortably possible.

Execution:

- Shrug your shoulders upward as high as possible.

- Pause briefly at the top.

- Lower slowly to the stretched position.

- Repeat for maximum repetitions.

HIT TIPS:

- Keep your arms straight when shrugging. Bending your arms involves your biceps.

- Focus on smooth, steady lifting and lowering.

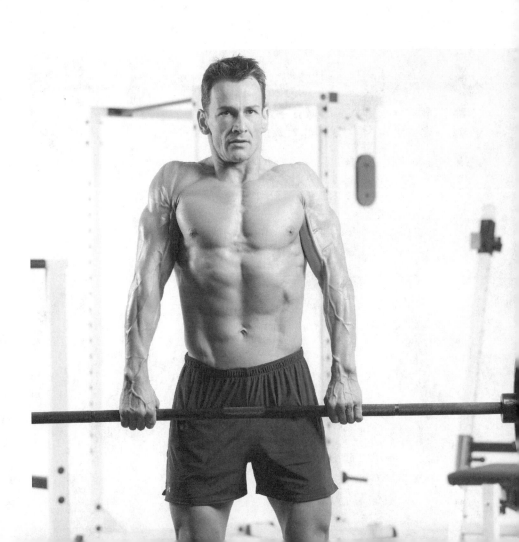

Next-Best Exercises

REVERSE CURL WITH BARBELL

Muscles Worked: Biceps, brachialis, and forearm extensors

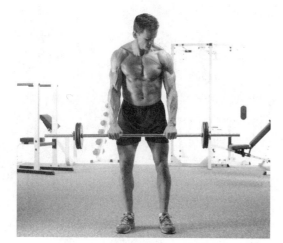

Start:

• Take a shoulder-width overhand grip on a barbell.

• Stand with your arms hanging at your sides.

• Keep your elbows against your sides throughout the exercise.

HIT TIPS:

• Practice strict form.

• Use a thick-handled bar for variety.

Execution:

• Curl the barbell smoothly to the top position. Do not move your elbows forward. Keep your hands in front of your elbows.

• Lower the bar slowly to the bottom.

• Repeat for maximum repetitions.

Next-Best Exercises

PUSHDOWN ON LAT MACHINE
Muscles Worked: Triceps

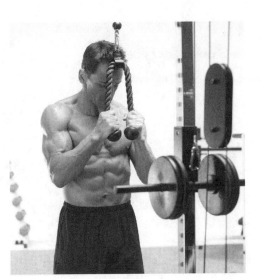

Start:

- Stand in a stable position in front of a lat machine with a neutral grip, which requires a rope attachment. If a rope is not available, use a straight-bar attachment at the top.

- Grasp the rope with a neutral, parallel grip. Your hands should be almost touching at the top.

- Pull your elbows to your sides and keep them there throughout the exercise.

HIT TIPS:

- Try various bars and grips. Some trainees like an underhand grip, and others like an overhand grip.

- Make the exercise harder by keeping your hands in front of your body.

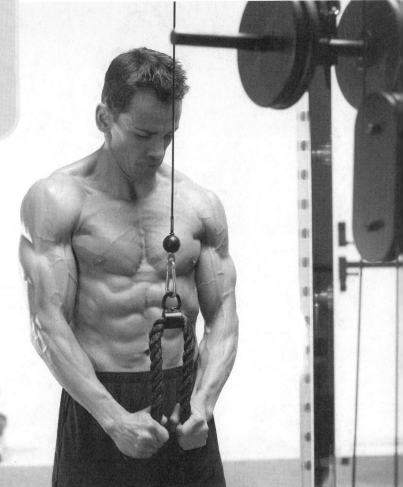

Execution:

- Push the rope handles toward the floor, keeping them under control.

- Keep your wrists stable, and don't lean forward. Let your triceps do the work.

- Pause when your arms are straight.

- Allow your hands to rise slowly until your elbows are comfortably bent.

- Repeat for maximum repetitions.

Next-Best Exercises

REVERSE WRIST CURL WITH BARBELL

Muscles Worked: Forearm extensors

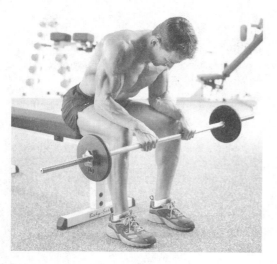

Start:

- Grasp a barbell with a palms-down grip.

- Rest your forearms on your thighs and sit down.

> **HIT TIPS:**
>
> - Do not move your shoulders or torso forward or backward. Keep them stable.
>
> - Use a light resistance initially.

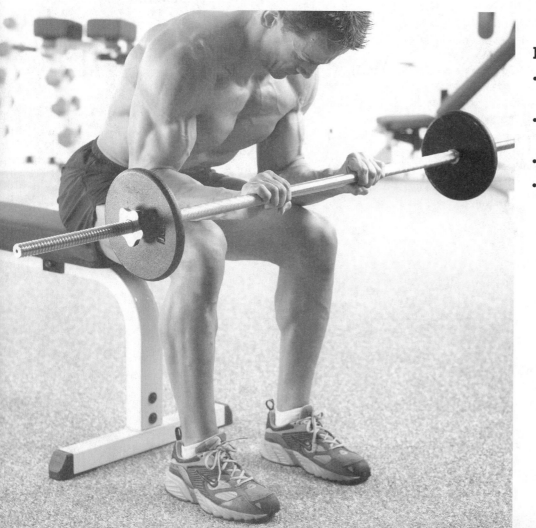

Execution:

- Curl the backs of your hands upward.

- Pause in the contracted position.

- Lower slowly to the bottom.

- Repeat for maximum repetitions.

Next-Best Exercises

PRONE BACK RAISE ON BENCH

Muscles Worked: Erector spinae and gluteus maximus

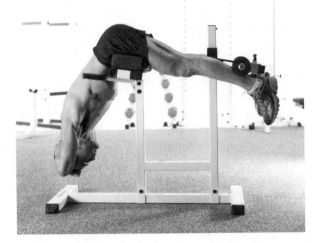

Start:

- Use a special back-raise bench (as shown), if possible, or have a partner assist you in this exercise.

- Lie facedown on a bench.

- Support the lower half of your body by having your navel even with the edge of the bench. Your partner should stand behind and hold your thighs and legs down.

- Place your hands behind your neck.

HIT HINTS:

- Make sure your navel area does not slide forward. Keep it at the edge of the bench.

- Do not move your head during the exercise. Keep it in one position.

Execution:

- Raise your torso backward smoothly. There should be a slight arch in your back in the top position.

- Lower your torso by bending at the waist.

- Make the turnaround at the bottom smoothly.

- Repeat for maximum repetitions.

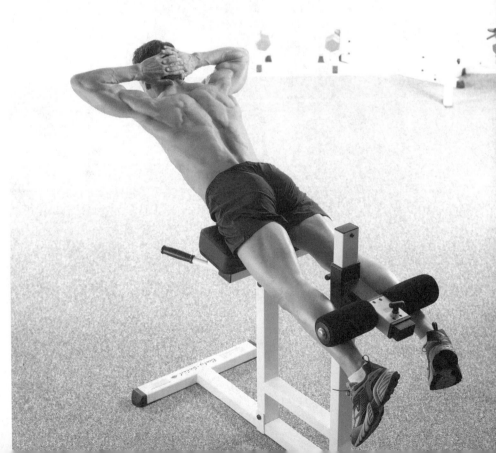

SIDE BEND WITH DUMBBELL

Muscles Worked: External and internal obliques

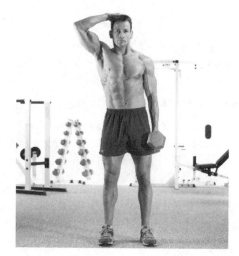

Start:

- Grasp a dumbbell in your left hand and stand erect.
- Position your feet shoulder width apart.
- Place your right hand on top of your head.

Execution:

- Bend laterally to your left as far as comfortably possible. At maximum stretch, try to reach even farther with your right arm and elbow.
- Return smoothly to the top-center position.
- Repeat for maximum repetitions.
- Switch the dumbbell to your right hand.
- Perform the side bend to your right side in a similar manner.

HIT TIPS:

- Do not let your shoulder drift forward or backward. Stay in the lateral plane.
- Stand tall each time you are in the top-center position.

Next-Best Exercises

REVERSE TRUNK CURL ON FLOOR

Muscles Worked: Rectus abdominis

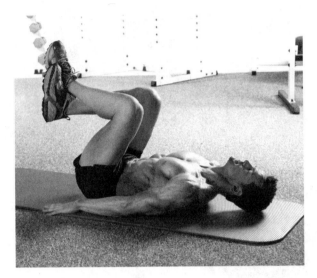

Start:

- Lie faceup on the floor with your hands on both sides of your hips.

- Bring your thighs up toward your chest so that your hips and knees are flexed. Cross your lower legs at your ankles.

HIT TIPS:

- Concentrate on curling your hips and thighs upward by contracting your abdominals only, rather than allowing momentum to assist you.

- Do not allow your legs to swing downward as you return to the bottom position. Keep your knees near your chest throughout the exercise.

Execution:

- Curl your hips toward your chest by lifting your buttocks and lower back off the floor. At the same time that you lift your buttocks, you must counterbalance your body by pushing down on the floor with your hands and arms.

- Pause briefly in the top position.

- Lower your hips slowly to the floor. Don't move your thighs and knees excessively. Keep them near your chest.

- Repeat for maximum repetitions.

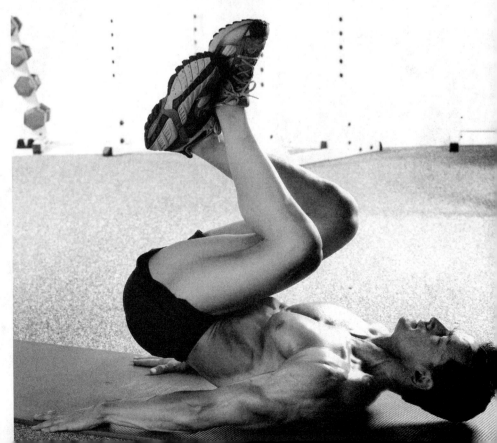

Chapter 14

BASIC ROUTINES FOR BEGINNERS AND INTERMEDIATES

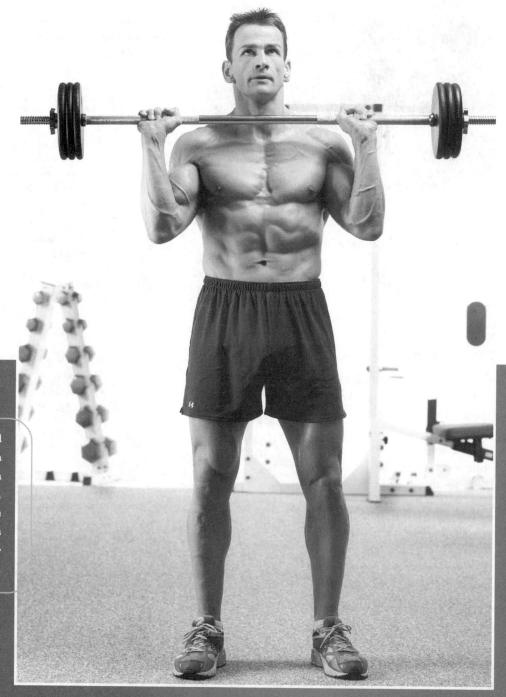

The overhead press is a basic, but often neglected, exercise for the major muscles of the shoulder girdle.

MANY LIFTERS FAIL to develop their muscles to anything close to their genetic potential, simply because they never learned the basics: basic guidelines + basic exercises + basic routines = a solid foundation. Without that foundation, such men usually default to multiple-set, high-volume exercise, which leads to overtraining, injuries, and poor results. Don't let yourself fall into that category. Take time to understand and apply the basic HIT routines before you move into the specialized and advanced programs.

First Things First

Here are some important things that you need to do before you start lifting.

Get a physical examination. If you haven't been to the doctor recently for a physical, now's the time to do it. Your doctor may find a problem that you didn't know you had, like high blood pressure, that would make a HIT program inappropriate for you. Or if you have preexisting problems with your knees, shoulders, and lower back, he may wave the caution flag. When you visit your doctor, bring this book, so he'll be able to see what you're about to undertake.

Make a workout card. You'll need to have a record card, similar to the one on page 237. In fact, you can make a photocopy of it and fill in the appropriate exercises in the left column. Then, simply write in your resistance and repetitions (in good form) across from the exercise and under the date. It's important to keep an accurate record of all your routines and workouts.

Consider a warmup and a cooldown. Evidence supports the need for a general warmup as a safeguard against injury. Almost any sequence of light calisthenic movements—such as head rotations, side bends, trunk twists, arm circles, and exaggerated walking in place—can precede a HIT workout. Three minutes of these movements (that's 3 *total* minutes, not 3 minutes of each) should be enough. You don't need to worry about specific warmups for individual muscle groups. The first 3 or 4 repetitions of each exercise take care of that.

You also need a brief cooldown after your workout. Just take about 3 minutes to walk around the workout area, get a big drink of water, and move your arms in slow circles. Doing so gradually shifts your mind and body into a more relaxed state.

Keep water handy for drinking. HIT can be dehydrating. Always have a plastic bottle filled with cold water handy so that you can drink between your exercises.

Routines for Beginners

First, some definitions.

To me, a beginner is either someone who is new to strength training or someone who knows his way around a gym but is new to HIT. After 24 weeks of training, a beginner becomes an intermediate. After another 24 weeks, or 48 total weeks of training, an intermediate moves to the advanced level.

With all beginner, intermediate, and advanced lifters, I like to work in 2-week and 6-week segments. Doing so makes the organization and record keeping simpler.

It's tough for a beginner to learn good exercise form and train intensely at the same time. So I recommend that beginners spend the first 2 weeks using lighter resistance and focusing more on learning the exercises.

HOW TO REDUCE HIT DURATION (NUMBER OF EXERCISES) AND FREQUENCY OVER 12 MONTHS

WEEKS	DAYS OF WEEK FOR 2 WEEKS[a]													
	M	T	W	T	F	S	S	M	T	W	T	F	S	S
	NUMBER OF EXERCISES													
1–2	8		8		8			10		12		12		
3–6	12		12		12			12		12		12		
7–12	12		12 NTF[b]		12			12		12		12		
13–18	12				12			12		12		12		
19–24[c]	12				12			12		12 NTF		12		
25–30	10				10			10		10 NTF		10		
31–36	10				10			10				10		
37–42	10				10 NTF			10				10		
43–48[c]	8				8 NTF			8				8		
49–54	8						8				8			

[a] Continue each 2-week segment for 6 weeks.

[b] NTF: Not to failure; stop 2 repetitions short of an all-out effort.

[c] After this 6-week segment, take a 9-day layoff.

Further, I think it's smart to start with a shorter list of exercises to learn. So I recommend that you do only exercises 1 to 8 the first week. On Monday of the second week, add two new exercises, then another two on Wednesday. On Friday of that second week, crank up the resistance and your intensity, but still don't go all out. At the beginning of the third week, you should be prepared to go to momentary muscular failure in good form.

I've created four routines for beginners. Each lasts 6 weeks. The heart of each routine is the 2-week training schedule, which you'll repeat three times. Remember what I explained in chapter 11: As you progress through the 6-week programs, you'll gradu-ally reduce your workout frequency from six times in 2 weeks to five times in 2 weeks, which includes a not-to-failure (NTF) workout. The chart shown above supplies an overall view of the reductions.

Beginning HIT Routine 1

1. Leg-curl machine

2. Leg-extension machine

3. Leg-press machine

4. Straight-arm pullover with one dumbbell

5. Bench press with barbell

6. Bent-over row with barbell

7. Overhead press with barbell

8. Biceps curl with barbell

9. Triceps extension with one dumbbell

10. Wrist curl with barbell

11. Standing-calf-raise machine

12. Trunk curl on floor

Remember, during the first week, to lighten the resistance and focus on performing exercises 1 to 8 with perfect form. During the second week, add exercises 9 and 10 on Monday, and exercises 11 and 12 on Wednesday. Practice moving closer and closer to failure, with heavier weights on each exercise. By the third week, you'll be ready to give each exercise your best effort.

Beginning HIT Routine 2

1. Leg-curl machine

2. Leg-extension machine

3. Leg-press machine

4. Standing-calf-raise machine

5. Bench press with barbell

6. Bent-over row with barbell

7. Lateral raise with dumbbells*

8. Shoulder shrug with barbell*

9. Bent-arm fly with dumbbells*

10. Triceps extension with one dumbbell

11. Biceps curl with barbell

12. Trunk curl on floor

*New exercise

You drop three exercises (straight-arm pullover, overhead press, and wrist curl), and you replace them with the lateral raise, shoulder shrug, and bent-arm fly. Remember that your first Wednesday workout of each 2-week segment will be not to failure (NTF).

Beginning HIT Routine 3

1. Squat with barbell*

2. Straight-arm pullover with one dumbbell

3. Stiff-legged deadlift with barbell*

4. Lateral raise with dumbbells

5. Bench press with barbell

6. Shoulder shrug with barbell

7. Bent-arm fly with dumbbells

8. Triceps extension with one dumbbell

9. Biceps curl with barbell

10. Wrist curl with barbell

11. Reverse trunk curl on floor*

12. Side bend with dumbbell*

*New exercise

Routine 3 introduces two great barbell exercises, the squat and the stiff-legged deadlift. Also, you'll add the reverse trunk curl and the side bend. You'll eliminate the leg curl, leg extension, leg press, and the bent-over row. During Routine 3, you'll reduce your frequency from 6 days in 2 weeks to 5 days. If you're following the chart, that means you skip the first Wednesday workout in each 2-week segment.

Beginning HIT Routine 4

1. Squat with barbell/Leg-press machine

2. Leg-curl machine

3. Leg-extension machine

4. Seated-calf-raise machine*

5. Bench press with barbell/Bent-arm fly with dumbbells

6. Shoulder shrug with barbell

7. Overhead press with barbell

8. Reverse curl with barbell*

9. Pushdown on lat machine*

10. Negative chinup*

11. Negative dip*

12. Reverse wrist curl with barbell*

*New exercise

Routine 4 brings six new exercises: seated calf raise, reverse curl, pushdown on lat machine, negative chinup, negative dip, and reverse wrist curl. You'll be dropping the straight-arm pullover, stiff-legged deadlift, lateral raise, triceps extension, biceps curl, wrist curl, and side bend. You'll notice there are two exercises listed in the number 1 and number 5 slots. Simply, this means that you alternate them. For example, do the squat on your first workout day, leg press on the second, squat on the third, and so on. During each 2-week segment, you'll train five times—but only four workouts will be HIT. One workout will be NTF. Don't forget

that as you get stronger, you must do less overall exercise.

Once you finish this 6-week program, you'll have completed 24 weeks of the basic HIT routines. You trained hard, you made significant progress, and you deserve a break. Please take a 9-day layoff from training. Rest, relax, and enjoy yourself. Then you'll be ready to move to the intermediate workouts.

Routines for Intermediates

I've created five intermediate routines. You'll follow a similar pattern to the one you used with the beginner routines, with gradual reductions in workout duration and frequency. Initially, you'll do five workouts in 2 weeks, with 10 exercises per workout. At the end of 24 weeks of intermediate work, you'll be doing three 8-exercise workouts in 2 weeks.

Intermediate HIT Routine 1

1. Leg-extension machine

2. Leg-curl machine

3. Squat with barbell

4. Standing-calf-raise machine

5. Bent-arm pullover with barbell*

6. Incline bench press with barbell*

7. Bent-over row with barbell

8. Triceps extension with one dumbbell

9. Biceps curl with barbell

10. Trunk curl on floor

*New exercise

You have two new exercises, the bent-arm pullover and the incline bench press. But you're still reducing your total exercises from 12 to 10 per workout. Notice that your Wednesday workout of the second week is NTF. The other four in each 2-week period are all-out efforts. After your 9-day layoff, you should be ready to pump some serious iron.

Intermediate HIT Routine 2

1. Leg-extension machine/Leg-curl machine

2. Stiff-legged deadlift with barbell/Leg-press machine

3. Standing-calf-raise machine/Seated-calf-raise machine

4. Bent-arm pullover with barbell/Straight-arm pullover with one dumbbell

5. Incline bench press with barbell/Bench press with barbell

6. Pulldown on lat machine*

7. Bent-over raise with dumbbells*

8. Triceps extension with one dumbbell/Biceps curl with barbell

9. Negative chinup/Negative dip

10. Side bend with dumbbell/Reverse trunk curl on floor

*New exercise

For the second intermediate routine, you'll stop doing the squat, bent-over row, and trunk curl, while adding the pulldown on lat machine and bent-over raise with dumbbells. The latter two are the only exercises you'll do each workout. You'll do the other exercises once each week. Because you're now on a twice-weekly schedule, you'll do one set of exercises on Monday, the other on Friday of each week.

Intermediate HIT Routine 3

1. Squat with barbell/Leg-press machine

2. Standing-calf-raise machine/Seated-calf-raise machine

3. Leg-extension machine/Leg-curl machine

4. Prone back raise on bench*/Stiff-legged deadlift with barbell

5. Pulldown on lat machine

6. Front raise with dumbbells*

7. Lateral raise with dumbbells/Bent-arm fly with dumbbells

8. Biceps curl with barbell/Triceps extension with one dumbbell

9. Bench press with barbell/Bent-over row with barbell

10. Four-way neck machine, front and back*/ Four-way neck machine, side to side*

*New exercise

You'll be adding the prone back raise, the front raise with dumbbells, and the four-way neck machine (if available). (The four-way neck is an optional exercise. If this machine is available in your gym, please ask for help in learning how to use it correctly.) Plus, as before, 8 of the 10 exercises are paired and alternated, so you'll continue to enjoy variety in your workouts. And one of your four workouts is NTF. Stay focused and train hard.

Intermediate HIT Routine 4

1. Leg-extension machine/Leg-curl machine

2. Leg-press machine

3. Standing-calf-raise machine

4. Stiff-legged deadlift with barbell

5. Straight-arm pullover with one dumbbell

6. Bench press with barbell/Overhead press with barbell

7. Negative chinup

8. Negative dip

No new exercises appear. You've effectively experienced them all, and you'll do fewer of them here—just eight per workout. As in the third intermediate routine, you'll do three HIT workouts and one NTF.

Intermediate HIT Routine 5

1. Leg-curl machine/Leg-extension machine

2. Squat with barbell/Leg-press machine

3. Standing-calf-raise machine/Seated-calf-raise machine

4. Bench press with barbell/Negative dip

5. Negative chinup/Biceps curl with barbell

6. Lateral raise with dumbbells/Bent-arm fly with dumbbells

7. Overhead press with barbell/Triceps extension with one dumbbell

8. Trunk curl on floor/Reverse trunk curl on floor

The last intermediate routine involves eight paired exercises, which once again are alternated back and forth into two workouts. You'll also drop the NTF workout and do just three HIT sessions every 2 weeks. During the sixth week of Routine 5, you should make a point to test yourself on four basic exercises: leg extension, leg press, bench press, and biceps curl. See how much weight you can lift for 10 strict repetitions. Then compare that number with what you did during the very first 2-week session. You should now be at least twice as strong on each of these four exercises.

In other words, if you did 125 pounds for 10 repetitions on the bench press during your initial 2-week period, you should now be able to do 250 pounds or more for 10 reps.

Chapter 15

ADVANCED TECHNIQUES: PUSH, PULL, AND SURPRISE

Heavy, negative-only dips are a tried-and-proven exercise to incorporate into your workouts.

EVERY LIFTER HOPES that tomorrow will bring a new technique that will somehow allow him to push, pull, and detonate his muscles to new growth. Most of this hope is wishful thinking and is, in part, promoted by the popular muscle magazines and their catchy, attention-getting headlines.

But instead of waiting for the new, bodybuilders would be better off looking for tried-and-true techniques from the past.

After 9 months to a year of consistent HIT, your rate of muscular growth does slow. But there are many techniques you can employ to change the nature of the pushing and pulling. Your goal is to surprise, rather than detonate, your muscles to new growth.

The major drawback of these advanced techniques is the increased likelihood of overtraining. Each of these techniques, when practiced properly, makes a greater inroad into your starting level of strength than does a normal HIT set. If you applied several at the same time, you could mess up the already delicate balancing act between inroad and recovery.

Here are the techniques I'll discuss.

- Cheating repetitions
- Forced repetitions
- Breakdown sets
- 1¼ repetitions
- Stage repetitions
- Pre-exhaustion sets
- Negative repetitions
- SuperSlow repetitions
- Extremely slow repetitions

Cheating Repetitions

This was the technique Arthur Jones used in chapter 1 to induce nausea during a set of biceps curls. The method could work for many exercises.

- Perform an exercise very strictly to momentary muscular failure.
- Use a little body momentum to get the weight past the sticking point on the positive phase. Lower the resistance in strict form.
- Use a little more body momentum to get the weight past the sticking point again, for 1 or 2 more repetitions.

Obviously, if this technique is not controlled, you could hurt yourself. Use it responsibly.

Forced Repetitions

Forced reps require a training partner.

- Select an exercise and do it to momentary muscular failure.
- Instruct your training partner to assist you ever so slightly on the positive phase so that you can get past the sticking point to the contracted position.
- Lower slowly on the negative phase.
- Do 1 or 2 more reps the same way.

Breakdown Sets

I've described this technique for use on a weight-stack machine, because that's the best equipment for it. You could also employ it with a barbell, although it's less practical. You'd have to have a spotter on both sides of the bar. You'll still need an assistant on a weight-stack machine, but it's a lot easier to find one than two.

- Select a weight you'd normally do for no more than 8 reps.

- Do the exercise to failure.

- Have the assistant, at your command, immediately pull the pin on the weight stack and place it in a weight about 20 percent lighter.

- Continue the exercise until you fail a second time. If you want, you can keep going that way for another set or two.

1¼ Repetitions

This works well if you feel you're weak in the final part of an exercise's range of motion.

- Start with a weight that's about 10 percent less than what you'd ordinarily use for 10 reps.

- Lift the weight to the contracted position and then pause.

- Lower the resistance a quarter of the way down and then lift it back to the top position. Pause again.

- Lower to the bottom and repeat, performing that extra quarter-rep each time you reach the contracted position.

You can also do the quarter-rep movement in the stretched position, but that should be done as part of a different set.

Stage Repetitions

Most exercises have a normal sticking point, where the resistance feels heavier than it does at other points. Likewise, when you near the lockout of any multiple-joint movement, the exercise feels easier. Stage repetitions help combat those heavier and lighter ranges.

- Divide the range of movement into thirds.

- Determine the hardest, next hardest, and easiest thirds, or stages, of the exercise.

- Start with a weight you can handle for 20 seconds in each stage, or 60 seconds for the entire set.

- Perform the hardest part first, the next hardest second, and the easiest last.

Pre-Exhaustion Sets

Arthur Jones applied pre-exhaustion sets with Casey Viator, Sergio Oliva, and many other bodybuilders whom he trained in the 1970s.

- Select related single-joint and multiple-joint exercises.

- Arrange the exercises, or machines, so that they're next to each other. It's important to move quickly from one exercise to the next.

- Perform the single-joint movement until failure.

- Get to the next exercise without delay.

- Perform the related multiple-joint exercise to failure.

The multiple-joint exercise brings into action surrounding muscle groups to force the pre-exhausted muscle to a deeper level of fatigue. Variations include switching the exercises (reverse pre-exhaustion) and adding a third exercise to the cycle (double pre-exhaustion).

A few practical examples: You might do a set of flies before chest presses, pre-exhausting your chest. Or you could do it in reverse, with the flies following the presses to reach a deeper level of fatigue in your pectorals. Finally, you could do flies and front raises before chest presses, thus pre-exhausting your pectorals and your front deltoids, leaving your triceps as the only fresh muscle group for the presses.

Negative Repetitions

Although not invented by Arthur Jones, he certainly popularized negative reps with his early writings and the design of his machines. Here are three ways to emphasize the negative.

Negative-Only Repetitions

• Find one or two training partners to assist you.

• Place 30 to 40 percent more weight on the barbell or machine than you'd normally use for 10 reps.

• Instruct your assistants to help you lift the resistance to the contracted position and smoothly transfer the load to you. *Note:* On chinups and dips, you can do without the spotters. All you need is a step placed underneath, and you can use your legs to climb to the top position.

• Lower the resistance slowly in 8 to 10 seconds. Try to feel each part of the range.

• Instruct your assistants to lift the weight quickly back to the contracted position.

• Repeat until you can no longer control, or guide, the resistance to the bottom.

Negative-Accentuated Repetitions

• Use an exercise machine that has a fused movement arm, as opposed to individual movement arms. No assistant is needed.

• Place 60 percent of the resistance on the machine that you'd normally use for 10 repetitions.

• Lift the movement arm into the contracted position with both limbs.

• Transfer the load to one limb. You now have 120 percent of what you could handle with one limb in a normal manner.

• Slowly lower the weight with one limb, taking 8 to 10 seconds.

• Raise the weight with both limbs and pause.

• Transfer the load to the other limb and slowly lower it.

• Continue alternating until you can no longer control it. Your goal is 6 negative-accentuated repetitions for each limb, or 12 repetitions altogether.

Forced-Negative Repetitions

• Find a training partner and use a machine that has a fused movement arm.

• Reduce the resistance that you'd normally handle for 10 repetitions by 30 percent.

• Lift the movement arm to the contracted position.

• Have your training partner push down on the resistance to increase the negative load. He can either push on the weight stack or the movement arm. In either case, he needs to do it smoothly, or he could do more harm than good. Also, if you're going to try this in a commercial gym, you might want to check with management first.

• Lower the movement arm in 8 to 10 seconds.

• Lift the movement arm back to the contracted position and repeat the forced negative.

• Stop when you can no longer guide the movement arm to the bottom.

SuperSlow Repetitions

SuperSlow is a trademarked training system developed by Ken Hutchins. The SuperSlow crowd believes that not enough attention is devoted to the performance of typical repetitions. As a consequence, momentum is often introduced into a set, which interferes with achieving the safest and best possible results. They recommend a 10-second positive and 10-second negative on each repetition, which makes the exercise harder. Although a training partner is not necessary for SuperSlow, it still helps to have someone count the seconds for you, at least during your first few SuperSlow workouts.

• Reduce the resistance by approximately 20 percent on each exercise. If you've used SuperSlow previously, you may not need to lighten the load.

• Cut your repetitions in half. Instead of performing 8 to 12, do 4 to 6.

• Concentrate on moving very slowly during the first and last 2 inches of the range of motion. Make the turnarounds smoothly.

• When you can't finish a repetition, continue pushing or pulling for another 5 to 10 seconds, even though the weight isn't going anywhere. Ease out of the repetition and move to the next exercise.

Extremely Slow Repetitions

Yes, you can go slower than SuperSlow. The idea is to move as slowly as possible on both the positive and the negative, while trying to avoid coming to complete stops during the repetition. (You will stop at certain points, but try to minimize it.) Exercises with a long range of movement work best.

• Experiment with various repetition goals. For example, you could try 15-second positives and 15-second negatives, with a maximum time limit of 120 seconds. That's 4 complete reps in 2 minutes.

• Keep the maximum time per set at 120 seconds.

• Try a 1-repetition set: for example, 30 seconds up and 30 seconds down in the chinup and dip. Or better yet, go for 60 seconds up and 60 seconds down.

Effective and Efficient Action

So now that you know about all these great techniques, you probably wonder how to use them. I'll show you in the next eight chapters, when I present specialized HIT routines for all your major muscle groups. This is advanced bodybuilding, which allows you to redesign your physique. You can focus on your thighs or specialize on weak calves. You can widen your back, broaden your shoulders, or deepen your chest. You can build more biceps peak or chisel your waist.

But you'll get the results you want only if you follow these rules.

• Perform the exercises exactly as described. If you must substitute a barbell exercise for a machine exercise, make sure they're similar.

• Do the specialized routine no more than four times in 2 weeks. In fact, very strong bodybuilders will probably get better results with three specialized workouts in 2 weeks. You must be the judge of your own best frequency.

• Ideally, use a specialized routine for 2 weeks. Three weeks is the absolute maximum. You can repeat the routine again after another 3 months of normal, nonspecialized training.

• Do at least 2 weeks of nonspecialized training in between each specialized routine. Don't go straight from one specialized routine to the next.

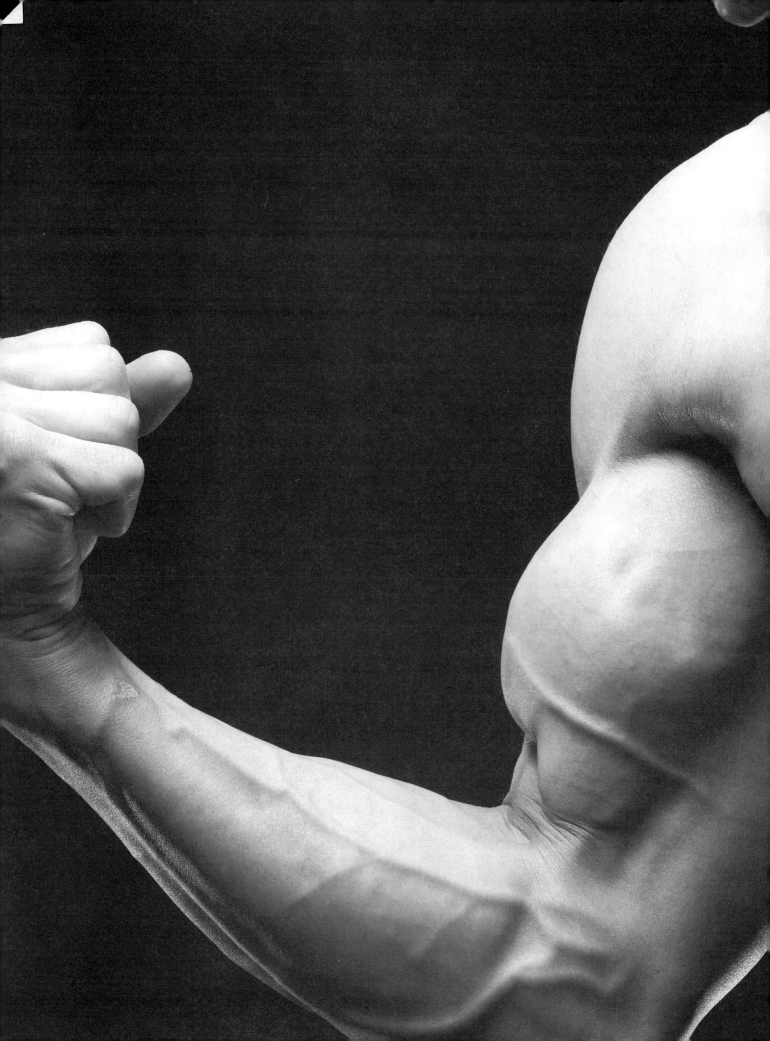

PART IV

SPECIALIZED HIT ROUTINES

Get ready to shock your thighs, inroad your shoulders, and stimulate your arms with the specialized HIT routines.

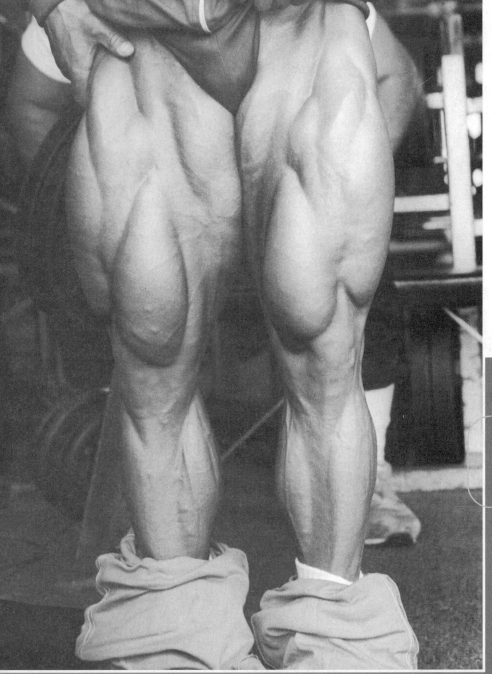

Chapter 16

HIPS AND THIGHS: SHOCKING YOUR STRONGEST MUSCLES

In the past 25 years, no bodybuilder has been able to top the thighs of Tom Platz.

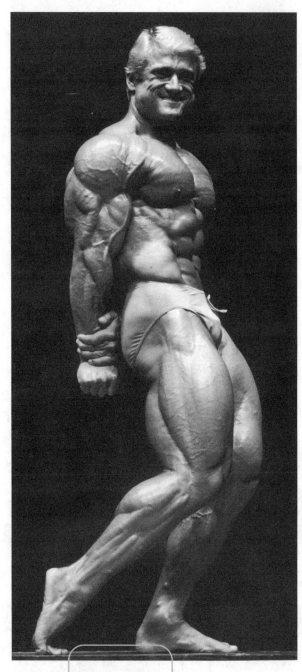

Check out the curve on Tom Platz's right hamstrings.

"THAT BUGGER TRAINS legs harder than anybody I've ever seen," Chris Lund, my British photographer friend, said to me during one of his initial visits to the Nautilus headquarters in the early 1980s. He noted that the bodybuilder he'd observed did squats with 500 pounds as if he were lifting 225. And we aren't talking a few ego-driven reps through a partial range of motion. These were deep squats—butt to calves—for 20 reps or more, sometimes going beyond failure. When this guy does squats or stiff-legged deadlifts, Lund said, "everybody in the gym just stops and stares. He's amazing."

The bodybuilder was Tom Platz, owner of the most unreal-looking quadriceps and hamstrings in the history of bodybuilding, and the guy who many thought should've won the Mr. Olympia in 1981.

I tell you this not to convince you to try full-range squats with 500 pounds. In fact, you shouldn't need to go nearly that heavy to get the results you want. My point is that the guy with the best leg-muscle development I've ever seen also trained his legs harder than anyone I've ever seen. In other words, there was a connection between his workouts and the results he got.

If you are stuck in a rut, this thigh routine just might get your legs growing again. Get ready for a shock.

The Thigh Cycle

The thigh cycle should be done exactly as described:

1. Leg extension, $1\frac{1}{4}$-repetition technique to failure, immediately followed by

2. Leg curl, 1¼-repetition technique to failure, immediately followed by

3. Leg press, extremely slow style: 4 repetitions in 120 seconds

Leg extension, 1¼-repetition technique: Sit in the leg-extension machine and place your feet behind the roller pads. Align the axis of rotation of the machine with your knees. Lean back and stabilize your body by grasping the handles or the sides of the machine. Straighten your legs smoothly. Pause. Lower one-quarter of the way down, then move back to the straight-legged position. Lower to the bottom and repeat the 1¼ technique for 8 to 12 repetitions or until momentary muscular failure. Go directly to the leg curl.

Leg curl, 1¼-repetition technique: Lie facedown on the machine and place your heels under the roller pads. Make certain that your knees are in line with the axis of rotation of the machine. Bend your knees and try to touch your heels to your buttocks. In the fully contracted position, come to a complete stop. Lower the resistance one-quarter of the way down, then return it to the contracted position. Lower slowly to the bottom. Repeat each 1¼ repetition 8 to 12 times.

The 1¼ extensions and curls both emphasize the contracted position of the involved muscles. The leg press, performed extremely slow, is going to work another range of the quadriceps, hamstrings, and buttocks.

Leg press, extremely slow, 4 repetitions in 120 seconds: You're in for a huge surprise on this exercise. If your gym's leg-press machine doesn't face a clock with a visible second hand, you'll need a stopwatch or a watch with a second hand that you can set up in plain sight. Or a training partner can talk you through each phase. Your goal is for each repetition to take 30 seconds: 15 seconds on the positive and 15 seconds on the negative, with no pausing at either end. The entire movement needs to be fluid and controlled. The exercise can be made easier by locking the knees at the end—but don't do it. In fact, if you can adjust your leg press by positioning the seat forward to limit the ending range of movement, you'll be better off. Use about half the weight that you'd normally lift on the leg press, at least for your initial workout.

Slide into the leg-press machine. Place your feet hip width apart on the foot pedal, stabilize your buttocks and torso, and begin the exercise as the second hand of the watch hits 12. Press slowly into the sliding platform or foot pedal. It need move only several inches during the first 5 seconds. At 10 seconds, you are just past the halfway mark, but remember, don't lock your knees. Doing so allows you to rest and makes the exercise easier. Near the lockout at 15 seconds, reverse direction and begin lowering in the same manner. Pay particular attention as you near the bottom turnaround. Stay focused and keep the tension and the movement smooth and slow.

The second repetition is harder than the first. The third repetition requires some concentrated attention on your breathing. Short belly breaths work best with the emphasis on blowing out rather than breathing in. Even with one-half of your normal leg-press resistance, you'll feel the fourth repetition throughout the entire range. That's it. Four repetitions in 120 seconds.

Keep Your Face Relaxed

Effective workouts require an all-out effort. If the by-product of this effort is excessive facial contortions and continual grunts and groans, the effort isn't as great as it could be.

Many small muscles of the face and neck contract when you grimace. This depletes a certain amount of energy. Relax all the uninvolved muscles, and you'll conserve the energy. That allows you to work the targeted muscles harder.

Making faces unnecessarily elevates your blood pressure. So does gritting your teeth and tightening your jaws. Because high-intensity exercise by itself elevates your blood pressure temporarily, there's no need to drive it higher by making faces.

Grunting results from straining to force out air while your mouth and nose are closed. This is called the Valsalva maneuver, which is potentially dangerous.

The stress and strain of lifting a heavy weight can produce this type of breathing. The resulting compressed exhalation dramatically increases pressure in the chest area, cutting down the volume of blood returning to the heart so drastically that dizziness or a blackout can result. There's even a possibility that blood vessels could rupture.

Some coaches instruct powerlifters to hold their breath, which creates a rigid rib cage and provides support for the upper spine. Though this may work for maximum single-repetition lifts, it's a bad idea for sets of 8 to 12 reps. And it's especially a bad idea for slow repetitions and negative-only sets.

Now imagine what it would feel like if, instead of cutting the weight in half, you would have reduced it by only 25 percent. Big, big difference. You probably would have failed on that fourth repetition. Well, that's what I want you to try during the next workout.

Thigh Specialization

I urge you to try this result-producing thigh cycle, but don't overdo it. Two or three cycles aren't better than one. Remember, it's the intensity of the exercise that stimulates muscle growth, not the amount of exercise.

Your maximum is two leg cycles a week for 2 weeks. Combine the three leg exercises of the cycle with five for your upper body. Choose from this list.

• Straight-arm pullover with one dumbbell

• Bench press with barbell

• Pulldown on lat machine

• Lateral raise with dumbbells

• Overhead press with barbell

• Shoulder shrug with barbell

• Biceps curl with barbell

• Triceps extension with one dumbbell

• Reverse curl with barbell

• Trunk curl on floor

Maximizing Results

It's important to remember that your body grows best by working it as an overall unit. If you want bigger thighs, you'll get them faster by working your upper body intensely as well. And the same concept holds true for specific upper-body goals you may have, as you'll see in subsequent chapters.

Chapter 17

CALVES:
"WORK 'EM AS HARD
AS YOUR ARMS!"

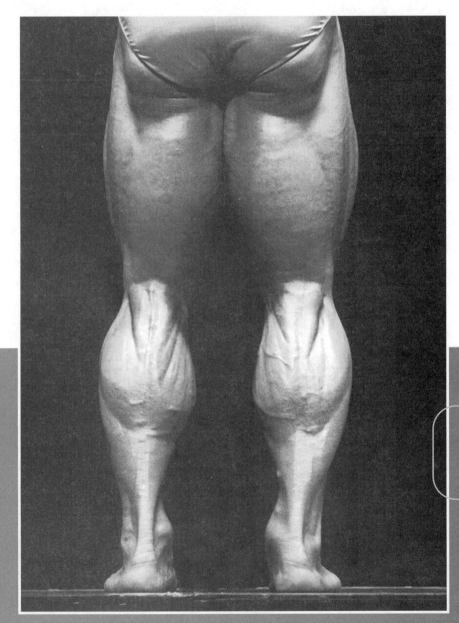

The contest lighting in this photo emphasizes perfectly Tom Platz's well-developed calves.

QUESTION: How did you get such great calves?

ANSWER: You want great calves? Simple. Work 'em as hard as your arms!

That question came from me at age 16. It was answered by John Gourgott, who was about to enter and win the 1960 Mr. Southern USA Contest. That was the first bodybuilding contest I'd ever seen, and I'd never talked to a man who was built like Gourgott. Let me digress a bit.

In the summer of 1959, three neighborhood buddies and I pooled our barbells and dumbbells in my parents' garage in Conroe, Texas. We figured that the more equipment we had, the faster we could all build our bodies. Combined, we had three barbells, six dumbbells, a flat bench with racks, and 300 pounds of plates. Our chinup bar was a limb on a medium-size sycamore tree in my front yard.

We all trained somewhat consistently for several months, even to the point of sending away to California for some tapered, black V-neck T-shirts. After training for 6 months, I weighed 155 pounds at a height of 5 feet 11 inches. The biggest of our group, Stuart Coyle, stood 6 feet 1 inch and weighed 170 pounds. Stu and I were the most motivated of the guys, as the others had pretty much lost interest. So we decided to drive 40 miles to the Downtown YMCA in Houston to attend the contest. We weren't disappointed.

Mr. Southern USA Contest

We arrived at the YMCA in time to observe the last part of the Olympic weight-lifting competition. In those days, most bodybuilding shows were held in conjunction with weight-lifting events. When we walked into the auditorium, there was a powerfully built man on stage performing a press overhead with 325 pounds. Stu and I were impressed. We had never seen anyone press 225 pounds, so 325 was indeed a thrill. The man's name was John Gourgott, and he was from New Orleans.

Gourgott was lean and muscular, and we figured he must be entered in the physique contest, too. At the conclusion of the lifting, Stu and I sneaked backstage and got a close look at the bodybuilders as they warmed up.

Our first sight was Gourgott stripped to his posing trunks performing one-arm chinups. He did 3 full repetitions with each arm. To this day, I've never seen another man as heavy—he weighed 196 pounds—who could do that.

I was fixated on Gourgott's arms, which were amazingly massive and muscular. But Stu kept telling me to check out Gourgott's calves, which were the biggest either of us had ever seen.

That's when we approached him, I asked him the question that leads off this chapter, and he gave us his formula.

Thirty minutes later, when it came time for Gourgott to pose, he bounded on stage, hit a double-biceps pose from the front, turned, and did the same pose from the back. He lowered his arms, turned slightly to one side, and pointed down with his right index finger to his left calf as the overhead spotlight illuminated it perfectly. Then, he slowly contracted his calf muscles . . . twice. And that was it—3 poses, and he was gone. All the other contestants had 10 or more poses.

"Man, that calf pose sealed it for John," Stu whispered as the next guy began his routine.

I said I wanted to see all the other poses I'd read

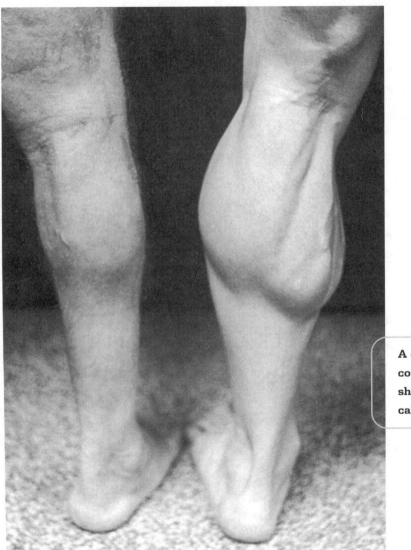

A dramatic comparison of short and long calf muscles.

about and seen in muscle magazines—side chest, lat spread, most muscular.

"Naw, man, it's best to keep the judges wanting more," Stu said. I'm sure he read that in a magazine, because this was the first contest either of us had ever attended.

Stu, though, was on to something. Gourgott indeed won first place. His career peaked in 1964, when he placed second in the Mr. America to Val Vasilef. (He'd added a few more poses by then.)

And Gourgott was on to something when he told us to train our calves as hard as our arms.

That means, in HIT workouts, you train them the same way you train your arms: with hard, brief exercise. The following routine will leave a lasting mark on your calves.

Advanced Calf Cycle

Do these three exercises back-to-back, with minimum rest in between.

1. Standing-calf-raise machine, immediately followed by

2. Bent-over calf raise on machine, immediately followed by

3. Bent-over calf raise on machine, stage repetitions

Standing-calf-raise machine: You'll need a calf-raise machine for this exercise. You can also use a barbell set up in a power rack. In that case, you'll need a sturdy 4-inch block or step to stand on to allow for a full range of movement.

Place the balls of your feet on the block or step. Raise your heels smoothly as high as possible. Attempt to go higher by standing on your big toes. Lower your heels slowly to the stretched position. Try to go lower by curling and spreading your toes. Repeat the movement for 12 repetitions. Move without resting to the bent-over calf raise.

Bent-over calf raise on machine: It's simple to go from the standing to the bent-over calf raise if you have a Nautilus multi-exercise machine. If you don't have that, many gyms now have specialized machines for this exercise. And if yours doesn't, you can always have a training partner sit across your back for what's called a donkey calf raise. Either way, you must follow the four-part protocol above: (1) raise your heels, (2) go up on your big toes,

(3) lower slowly, and (4) curl and spread your toes. Repeat until momentary muscular failure.

At this point, there's a little trick that you must do before going to the next exercise. Quickly raise one foot and shake it for 2 seconds. Do the same thing for your other foot. The entire pause/shake should take no more than 6 seconds. Then get back to the bent-over calf-raise position.

Bent-over calf raise on machine, stage repetitions: Divide the calf raise into equal stages: top, middle, and bottom. Go for 20 seconds in the top third of the range of motion. Do these partial movements slowly, and try to get up on your big toes. After 20 seconds, do the middle third of the range for another 20 seconds. Finally, do 20 seconds in the bottom, stretched position.

Your calves will feel a deep burn from this cycle. That's okay; work through it. Within 3 minutes of finishing this routine, your calves should be pumped more than an inch larger than normal. That means growth.

Other Exercises and Frequency

Same rules as before: Do this calf cycle four times in 2 weeks, maximum. The rest of your workout should include five other exercises, one for your thighs and four for your upper body.

After 2 weeks, back off and let those calves grow. You can return to the calf cycle after 3 months.

Chapter 18

UPPER BACK:
THE POSITIVE EFFECTS
OF DIRECT NEGATIVES

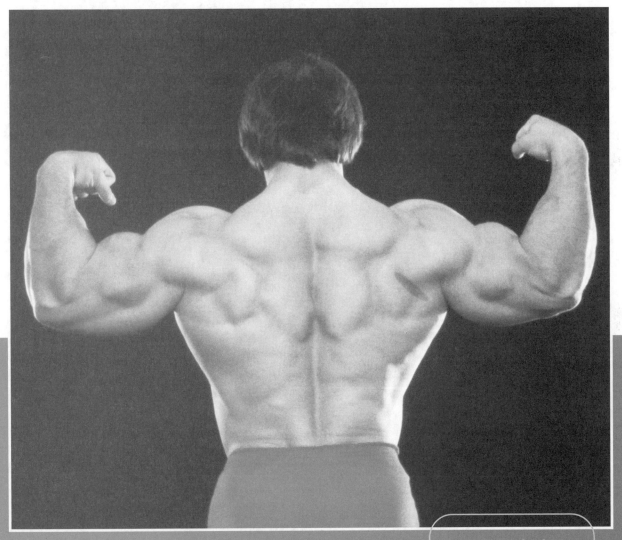

Casey Viator displays
his muscular upper-back
development.

THE FOREMOST MUSCLE of the back is the latissimus dorsi. This muscle joins the lower part of the spine and sweeps up the armpit, where it inserts into the upper-arm bone. When the latissimus dorsi muscles contract, they pull the upper arms from an overhead position down to the sides.

Traditionally, when lifters hit their lats with barbells and dumbbells, they do pullovers or bent-over rows. With access to a lat machine, they'll do pulldowns to the chest or behind the neck.

But there's a problem: All these exercises require the lifter to hold on to the barbell, dumbbells, or various bars with his hands. As a result, the smaller, weaker arm muscles tire before the larger, stronger latissimus dorsi muscles are fully overloaded. That's why Arthur Jones worked for more than 20 years to build a good pullover machine. This machine bypassed the hands and forearms and placed the resistance directly on the body part that was moved by the lats: the upper arms. All these years later, I still don't think anyone has invented an exercise or machine that surpasses the Nautilus-type pullover machines for helping you achieve full development of your lat muscles.

The Creator's Favorite Lat Routine

Jones and Casey Viator had a simple two-exercise lat routine, which they both used during the early 1970s.

1. Pullover machine, negative accentuated or negative only, immediately followed by

2. Chinup, negative only

Pullover machine, negative accentuated or negative only: Jones much preferred the negative-

The Gripping Truth about Pulldowns and Chinups

The latissimus dorsi are the largest, strongest muscles of the upper body. When highly developed, they add impressive width and thickness not only to your upper back but also to your overall chest size.

Many bodybuilders, however, fail to completely develop these muscles. More often than not, this occurs because they use the wrong hand spacing and grip.

One common mistake is using a wide grip on lat pulldowns and pullups. Bodybuilders believe that wide hand spacing provides more stretch and a greater range of movement for the lats. But the truth is the opposite: A wide grip provides *less* stretch for the lats than you'd get with a narrow grip. Furthermore, the wide grip actually prevents a greater range of movement by allowing the upper arms less rotation at the shoulder joints.

Now let's look at grip. Your biceps are strongest when your hands are supinated—turned toward you. Yet most bodybuilders work their lats with their hands pronated—turned away from them—which puts them at their weakest. Since the biceps are important supporting muscles for the lats, you'll be able to work your lats harder if you use a supinated grip when you do chinups.

Understanding the specific actions of your major muscles is a vital step toward efficient bodybuilding. Don't fall into the trap of doing an exercise because you like it, or avoiding an exercise because it's difficult. In general, the harder an exercise, the better the results. As an efficient bodybuilder, you should not look for ways to make exercises easier. Look for ways to make them harder, and thus more productive.

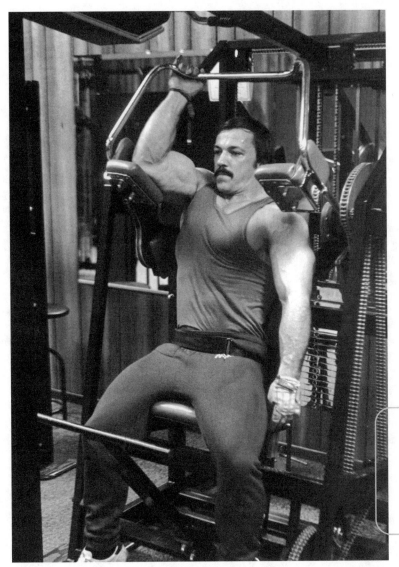

Pullover machine,
negative accentuated:
The idea is to pull the
padded bar over with
both arms and lower
with only one arm.

accentuated style during his personal training. This is where you take 60 to 70 percent of your normal 10-repetition resistance and use two arms on the positive and then alternate between a negative with the right arm and a negative with the left arm. With the proper resistance, you should just be able to get 12 positive repetitions with both arms and 6 negative repetitions with each arm.

Viator's negative-only pullovers required strong helpers to stand on both sides of the movement arm. He'd use the entire weight stack—and often added another 25 to 50 pounds. The assistants' job was to help Viator get into the fully contracted position. Then they'd transfer the resistance to his arms, and he'd perform a slow negative in 8 to 10 seconds. Eight slow negative repetitions didn't just wipe out the bodybuilder, it exhausted the spotters as well.

If you don't have access to a Nautilus-style pullover machine, you'll have to make do with a heavy, bent-arm pullover with a barbell.

Chinup, negative only: Go straight from the pullover to whatever station or machine you're going to use for negative-only chinups with added resistance. The Nautilus multi-exercise machine, if you have one in your gym, is perfect. Add about 50 pounds to the movement arm if you're reasonably strong. Slip into the padded belt, climb the steps until your chin is above the crossbar, hold on to the bar with an underhand grip, pause with your elbows tucked close to your body, ease your feet off the steps, bend your knees, and slowly lower yourself, using only your arms to resist gravity.

When you reach the bottom, climb quickly back to the top and repeat the slow negatives for at least 6 repetitions. Because your lats are pre-exhausted, your hands and biceps are temporarily stronger than them now. So you should be able to get a deep in-road into your lat strength.

If you can't get at least 6 reps, slip out of the

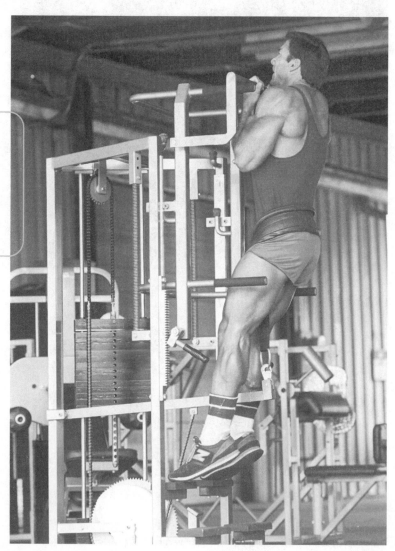

With 120 pounds attached around his waist, Boyer Coe has climbed into the top position of a negative chinup and is prepared to do a slow lowering repetition.

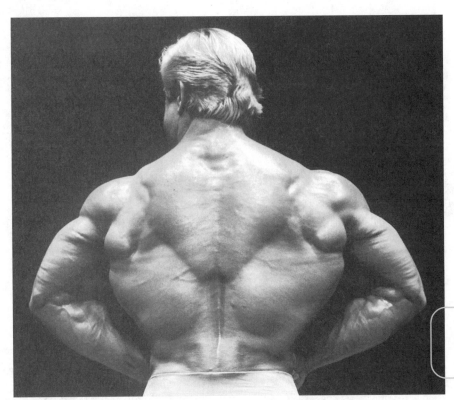

Tom Platz contracts his thick upper back and wide lats.

belt and do several negative repetitions with only your body weight.

That's it for your lats: only two negative exercises. Afterward, however, it will feel as if all the blood in your body is being directed to your lats. Get a cold drink of water, rest a few minutes, and ready yourself for six other exercises for the rest of your body, which should be performed in the four-times-in-2-weeks manner. It's your choice on the selection and the order, but here's a suggestion.

• Pullover machine, negative accentuated or negative only

• Chinup, negative only

• Lateral raise with dumbbells

• Bench press with barbell

• Shoulder shrug with barbell

• Leg-extension machine

• Stiff-legged deadlift with barbell

• Side bend with dumbbell

Lats Wider Than Your Shoulders

Arthur Jones always said that the potential size of the lats was far out of proportion to the maximum size of similar muscle groups. So great, in fact, that he often said it was possible to build lats wider than your shoulders.

The key was the stimulation power of the resistance being applied directly to the upper arms through the elbows. Remember that stimulation power as you focus intensely on those negative pullovers.

Feel your lats moving out and beyond your shoulders. It could happen to you.

Chapter 19

SHOULDERS AND NECK:
HOW TO DRESS FOR SUCCESS

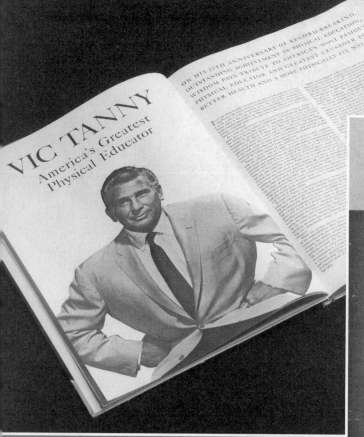

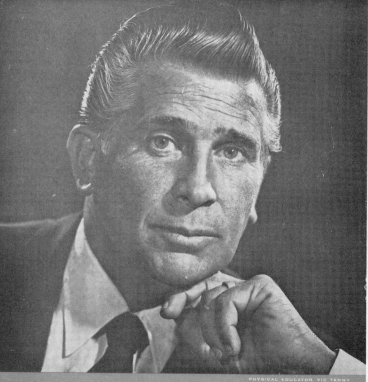

As shown in the May 1961 issue of *Wisdom* magazine, Vic Tanny's broad shoulders and full neck were the picture of strength, vitality, and confidence. In the early 1930s, Tanny won the New York State weight-lifting championship.

IN THE 1950s and 1960s, Vic Tanny was one of the few bodybuilders to evolve into a successful businessman. For many years, he had a penthouse apartment in New York City. He had a very profitable chain of fitness centers throughout the United States and had been involved in a number of multi-million-dollar deals. That meant that he, the bodybuilder, had to put on a suit, get into a boardroom with a bunch of other guys in suits, and convince them to make whatever deal was on the table at the moment. His secret to success, he told me one day in 1982, was the size of his shoulders and neck.

"Picture a mahogany boardroom table that is surrounded by a dozen fine leather chairs. Seated in those leather chairs are Wall Street—type power brokers and executives dressed in coats and ties. When you get too many powerful people together, almost everyone becomes self-centered and cautious. How you look from the chest up—because that's all anyone can see from a seated position—makes major impact.

"I know I've shouldered and necked more of my ideas across than I've talked through with reason."

Tanny added that he always hired guys with muscular necks to manage his health clubs. "I never went wrong with them. I've been all over the world and experienced almost everything, and I know that nothing sets a man apart like wide shoulders and a full neck."

Necksophilia

You can disguise your waistline in a suit. But you can't hide your shoulders and your neck. Muscle atrophy first shows up in your deltoids, trapezius, and neck muscles. You may not notice shrinkage in your biceps and triceps, but if your "yoke" muscles shrink, your shirts and suits will fit differently. And maybe, if Tanny is right, people will take you a little less seriously.

In other words, dressing for success begins beneath your coat and tie.

Fortunately, your shoulders and neck are some of the easiest muscles to develop.

The Shoulder and Neck Routine

My recommended workout is a bit different from other specialized routines in that I want you to work your shoulders at the start of the workout, and your neck and trapezius at the end. Although I list 11 exercises here, you're really doing 8. Three of the exercises are breakdown sets of the preceding movement.

1. Lateral raise, then decrease weight by 20 percent and move to

2. Lateral raise to failure

3. Overhead press, then decrease weight by 20 percent and move to

4. Overhead press to failure

5. Leg-curl machine

6. Leg-extension machine

7. Pullover

8. Pulldown on lat machine

9. Four-way neck: back, front, sides

10. Shoulder shrug with barbell, then decrease weight by 20 percent and move to

11. Shoulder shrug to failure

America's Greatest Crusader for Health and Fitness

When Vic Tanny decided to move to Daytona Beach, Florida, in the early 1980s, I gained a great friend. Tanny and I spent countless hours over the next few years discussing training, the fitness business, and his adventures as a world traveler.

His name isn't as famous as it once was, but here's what he accomplished.

• In the summer of 1940, he started what was perhaps the first modern fitness center in the United States, in Santa Monica, California.

• He claimed he built the first-ever bench-press rack in 1940 for that gym.

• Tanny wrote a successful column for *Strength and Health* magazine during the 1940s that helped to popularize the famous outdoor training area in California called Muscle Beach.

• He owned and operated more than 100 Vic Tanny Health Centers throughout the United States during the 1950s and 1960s. Tanny's clubs eventually merged with other groups to become the Health & Tennis Corporation of America in Chicago and New York, and the Holiday Spa in California. Most of these clubs are now part of the Bally Total Fitness chain.

• He was featured on the cover of the May 1961 issue of *Wisdom* magazine, in which he was labeled "America's Greatest Physical Educator."

• His younger brother, Armand Tanny, was a champion bodybuilder in the 1950s and today is a feature writer for *Muscle & Fitness*. Vic's son, Vic Tanny Jr., was also involved in bodybuilding competitions, in the 1970s.

I lost a great friend when Tanny died in 1985. He was never too busy to spend time with me or, for that matter, anyone interested in the fitness business. Thanks, Vic!

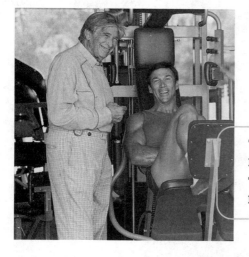

This photo of Vic Tanny with Boyer Coe was snapped while Tanny was visiting the Nautilus headquarters in 1983.

Lateral raise, breakdown set: Use dumbbells or a lateral-raise machine for this movement. I prefer the machine. Regardless of the tool available, your goal is to target your middle deltoid. Most trainees use more of their front deltoids in this exercise than they do the middle sections. To understand why, and how to correct this situation, let's examine the deltoid.

The deltoid is a triangular muscle that drapes over the shoulder joint with one angle pointing down the arm and the other two bent around the front and back of the shoulder. The deltoid muscle divides into three sections: front, side, and back. The front section usually covers the largest surface area, sometimes as much as 50 percent of the fibers of the deltoid. The middle amounts to 35 percent, and the back section takes up the remaining 15 percent. The middle deltoid, when significantly developed, provides dramatic width to your shoulders.

To target the middle deltoid, your upper arm must move not only to the side but also slightly back. What do most guys do? They move to the side, yes, but they raise the upper arm slightly to the front. Thus, after a repetition or two, they are using as much front deltoid as they are middle deltoid.

The idea is to angle your upper arms slightly behind your torso as you raise them laterally. You can accomplish this best by leaning 20 degrees forward from your waist as your arms move up. You won't be able to handle as much resistance as you usually do, but you'll be working your middle deltoid to a much greater extent. With a little practice, you'll get the hang of this unique version of a traditional exercise.

Either standing with dumbbells or seated in the lateral-raise machine, lean forward 20 degrees. Stay in this leaning-forward position throughout the exercise. Lift your upper arms to about chin level. Pause at the top. Lower slowly to the bottom. Resist the temptation to lean backward. Keep the movement smooth at all times. If you're using dumbbells, keep your elbows locked and the weights on the dumbbells parallel to the floor throughout the movement. In other words, don't let one side of the dumbbell tilt forward or backward. It should remain straight.

Do as many repetitions as possible in good

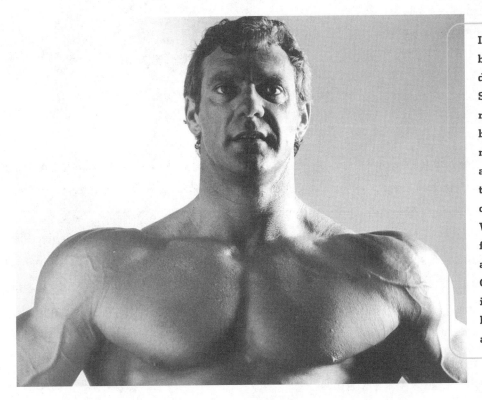

In professional bodybuilding circles during the 1980s, Scott Wilson was recognized for his broad shoulders and massive deltoids. Just after this photo was taken, I measured with calipers the width of Wilson's shoulders, from deltoid to deltoid, at exactly 24 inches. Only a handful of men in the world today have shoulders that are 2 feet across.

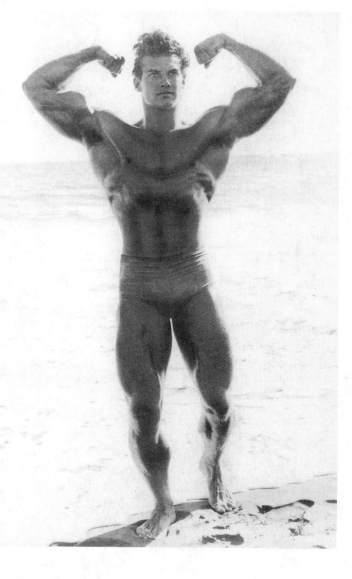

Steve Reeves, at age 21, won the Mr. America in 1947. "The first time I saw Steve," Vic Tanny remembered, "he was walking near the water at the Santa Monica Pier. People all over the beach were staring and pointing. About 50 yards away, some of us were practicing our lifts, and as he approached, I couldn't take my eyes off his shoulders. They were the broadest and most impressive I've ever seen."

form. After the last repetition, reduce the resistance by 20 percent and immediately do a second set of the lateral raise. Again, resist the desire you'll have to move your upper arms forward and bring into action your front deltoids. Remember, you want to fatigue your middle deltoids. Do as many repetitions as possible of this second set.

Overhead press, breakdown set: Your deltoids should already be fatigued as you progress to the press. That's good. You're going to use your triceps, which haven't been worked, to force your exhausted deltoids to a deeper level of fatigue. So move quickly to the press.

Use a barbell or an overhead-press machine for this exercise. Take less weight than you normally select. Your hands should be shoulder width apart. Press the weight over your head. Don't lock your elbows. Keep a slight bend in them. Lower the weight slowly back to your upper chest and then repeat.

When you can no longer complete a full repetition in good form, stop the movement. Quickly reduce the resistance by 20 percent. Do a second set in the same style as the first. Afterward, your shoulders should feel as though someone seared them with a blowtorch, and your pump should be extraordinary.

Leg curl and leg extension: Do smooth, slow sets of the leg-curl and leg-extension machines. Be sure to pause in the contracted position of each exercise. If you don't have access to these machines, then you may substitute the barbell squat or the leg press.

Pullover and pulldown: Again, I prefer machines for these two movements. If the machines aren't available, try the straight-arm pullover with a dumbbell and the bent-over row with a barbell.

Four-way neck: Nautilus makes the best neck machine on the market. If you have it available, use it. Hammer and MedX also have four-way neck machines that work well. Without a neck machine, you'll have to employ a neck harness in all four directions: back, front, right side, and left side. Or it's possible to get a neck workout by lying on a bench and having a partner supply hand/arm resistance to your moving head (see the neck exercise question in chapter 30 on page 226). Keep your movements slow and deliberate.

Shoulder shrug, breakdown set: Nautilus makes a shoulder-shrug machine that targets your traps. So does Hammer. If you can't find either, then use a heavy barbell or dumbbells. Stand erect with the barbell in front of your thighs. Raise your shoulders as high as possible; try to touch them to your ears. Pause. Don't roll your shoulders backward or forward. Lift them in a vertical line. Don't bend your arms. Lower your shoulders slowly to the stretched position. Repeat for maximum repetitions.

Immediately decrease the resistance by 20 percent. Do a second set of shoulder shrugs to muscular failure. And keep your form strict.

Holding the Trump Cards

I can close my eyes and still see Vic Tanny, with his dominant wisdom, repeating the following:

"Broad shoulders and a big neck. You need them both . . . if you're going to be successful in the business world."

I feel certain that Tanny, in his prime, would have been able to swing almost any deal his way, even if it involved competing with Donald Trump. Why? Because Tanny would have had the very best trump cards: wide shoulders and a full, muscular neck.

Chapter 20

CHEST: POWERFUL PECTORALS

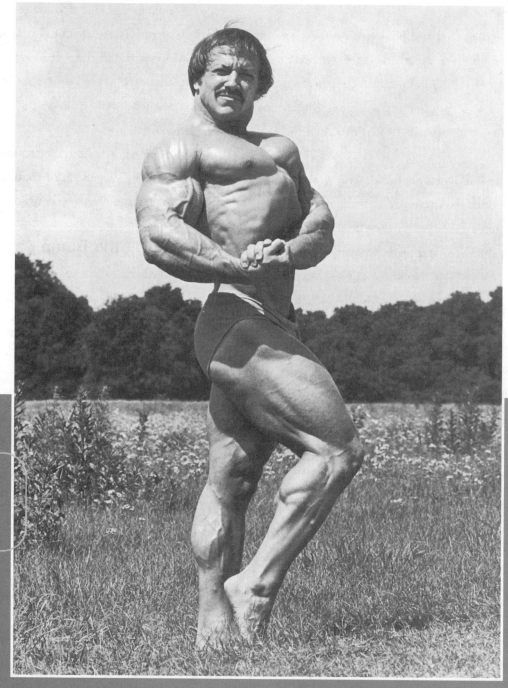

A large rib cage and thick pectorals equal Casey Viator.

IN CHAPTER 17, I mentioned attending my first bodybuilding show in Houston, Texas, and being impressed with the massive arms and calves of the winner, John Gourgott. Two years later, in the spring of 1962, I was about to enter my first contest.

It was my senior year at Conroe High School, and even though I played on the football, basketball, and baseball teams, I managed to continue weight training once or twice a week. It showed, too; my body weight had gone from 155 to 190 pounds in 2 years. All the original guys who'd trained with me in my parents' garage had moved on, which means I'd inherited all their weights (along with a lot more from guys around town who were briefly interested in the iron game).

I signed up for both the weight-lifting and the bodybuilding competitions at the Southwest YMCA in Houston. It was for teenagers only, and because Gourgott had entered both events in the 1960 show, I thought, "Why not?"

The day started off pretty well. Even though I'd never used an Olympic barbell set, I managed to press 180 pounds, snatch 135, and clean-and-jerk 200. That was good enough for second place in the light-heavyweight division.

Later, in the warmup room prior to the bodybuilding show, I met a competitor who had the biggest, thickest pectoral muscles I ever saw, before or since. That's right: bigger than Gourgott's, Viator's, and Oliva's, proportionately speaking.

The owner of those pecs was Ronnie Ray of Dallas. At a little over 5 feet tall, Ray weighed 150 pounds—and it was mostly pecs and upper body. It's not that his legs were undeveloped. But his pectorals, triceps, and biceps were so thick that he looked distorted. He told me that in 1961, while weighing 140 pounds, he had won a national YMCA chinup contest by doing 33 chins.

I thought Ray should've won, but he finished second. I got third place. It was the start of a great friendship (not to mention two pretty good careers). We crossed paths at weight-lifting and bodybuilding competitions throughout Texas and Oklahoma over the next decade.

Strength, Size, and Form

It was an interesting time to compete, in that lifting and physique contests were still held in conjunction with each other. Besides competing in Olympic-style lifting—which included the press, snatch, and clean and jerk—you could enter the "odd lifts" contest. Powerlifting was not yet recognized as an official AAU sport, so this was the next best thing. The odd lifts were the bench press, squat, deadlift, curl, and upright row.

Ray and I usually entered the odd lifts and bodybuilding competitions.

His specialty was the bench press. In fact, in the first contest we entered at the Tulsa, Oklahoma, YMCA, he benched more than he squatted or deadlifted. Several years later, however, that wasn't the case. Ray worked hard on the squat and deadlift and became a consistent winner in both. As soon as powerlifting became an AAU sport, he was the overall national champion in the 181-pound class. He went on to establish American and world records in the bench press, lifting well over 500 pounds and weighing less than 200 pounds.

But what was perhaps most impressive about Ray was his form. Whether he was training or going

Muscular Contraction: All or Nothing!

Individual muscle fibers perform on an all-or-nothing basis. Only the number of fibers that are actually required to move a particular amount of resistance are involved in any movement.

In effect, a fiber is working as hard as possible or not at all. A movement against light resistance doesn't involve a small amount of work from all the fibers in the muscles contributing to this movement. It's the opposite: Minimal fibers are involved—the fewest your body needs to move the weight—but they're working as hard as possible at that moment.

One individual fiber may be involved in each of several repetitions in a set of an exercise, but it won't contribute an equal power to each repetition. The fiber will always work as hard as possible—if it works at all—but its strength will decline with each additional repetition.

A set might work this way: The first repetition involves 10 fibers, with each fiber contributing 10 units of power to the movement. The second repetition involves the same 10 fibers, which then contribute only 9 units of power each, and one previously uninvolved fiber. That fresh fiber, the 11th one, contributes 10 units of power, bringing the total power production up to the same level as that involved in the first repetition.

The third repetition might involve the original 10 fibers, with each of them now contributing only 8.1 units of power. The 11th fiber is still in the mix, but now it's only contributing 9 units of power. So a 12th fiber comes is, and that one contributes 10 units of power.

Each of the first 3 repetitions, therefore, would result in exactly the same amount of power production. And all the involved fibers would always be contributing to the limit of their momentary ability. (In other words, they're doing all they can at the moment they're forced to do it.) The fibers, however, would not be contributing equally, and the actual number of involved fibers would change from repetition to repetition.

To produce significant growth stimulation, the set must be continued to a point where as many fibers have been involved as possible, and where at least some of the fibers have been worked to momentary failure.

for a world record, every repetition was performed in the absolute strictest style. Most of his competitors would use any tactic they could get away with—bouncing the bar off their chests or short-ranging the squat—but Ray refused to compromise. He always exceeded the requirements in the rule book.

His bench presses were a work of art. I've seen him do 400 pounds for 6 strict repetitions—and he paused with the bar on his chest for a full 10 seconds before each movement. Furthermore, many of his repetitions were done in an extremely slow style.

In my opinion, Ray's tremendous pectorals and overall body strength were a result of his excellent form on every exercise. If you want a massive chest, take a tip from Ronnie Ray and pay particular attention to feeling the resistance in each point throughout the range of movement in all your repetitions. This certainly makes the exercise harder, but it also makes it more productive.

Powerful Pectoral Routine

The four-exercise chest cycle is brutal.

1. Bent-arm fly with dumbbells, immediately followed by

2. Bench press with barbell, breakdown set, immediately followed by

3. Dip, negative only

4. Pushup on floor, negative only

Bent-arm fly with dumbbells: Grasp two heavy dumbbells, sit on a narrow bench, lie back, and press the dumbbells over your chest. Lower the dumbbells slowly to the sides of your chest. Keep your hands, elbows, and shoulders in line. Stretch in the bottom and then smoothly move the dumbbells back to the top position. Repeat for 8 to 12 repetitions or until failure. Sit up, place the dumbbells on the floor, and move to the bench press.

Bench press with barbell, breakdown set: You'll need 20 percent less resistance on this exercise than you normally use for 10 repetitions. Also, you'll need to prepare the barbell for one breakdown by leaving the collars off and having some small plates for quick removal at each end. The breakdown should be approximately 20 percent of the weight on the bar, or 10 percent from each end. And you'll need a training partner on each side to strip the weight off the barbell after the first set.

Grasp the barbell slightly wider than shoulder width and bring it to arm's length over your chest. Lower the barbell slowly, touch your chest, and press the bar smoothly to the top position. Repeat for maximum repetitions. On the last repetition, pause in the top position and have the two assistants remove 10 percent from each end of the barbell. Continue performing slow, smooth repetitions until positive failure. Have your spotters help you

replace the bar on the racks and instantly move to the parallel bars for dips.

Dip, negative only: The bent-arm fly and the bench press should have thoroughly pre-exhausted your pectorals. The dip, performed in a negative-only manner, will use your triceps to force your pectorals to work even harder.

Place a chair or sturdy box between the dip bars (or use a Nautilus multi-exercise machine). Climb to the top position. Straighten your arms, remove your feet from the chair, and stabilize your body. Lower slowly to the stretched position. The negative movement should take a full 8 seconds. Climb back quickly to the top and repeat for 8 to 12 repetitions. If you can perform more than 12 repetitions, you'll need to add resistance (strap on a waist belt and attach a weight plate or dumbbell to the chain).

Pushup on floor, negative only: You won't feel like doing pushups after dips; in fact, you may not be able to do even one. But give them a try anyway. With your hands directly under your shoulders, do as many pushups as you can in a normal fashion. Then, do several more in a negative-only manner by using your knees to assist you in getting into the locked-out position. Slowly lower your chest to the floor.

Adding to the Chest Cycle

I recommend adding these exercises to complete your workout.

- Bent-over row with barbell/Biceps curl with barbell
- Trunk curl on floor
- Standing-calf-raise machine
- Squat with barbell

Size and Thickness

I remember watching Ronnie Ray do dumbbell bench presses one afternoon in his Dallas club, and it took four people to hand him his weights. Why? Because each dumbbell weighed 140 pounds!

After watching him perform that exercise with perfect form for 8 repetitions, and noticing that afterward his chest appeared to be about 18 inches thick, I made up my mind that during my next workout I was going to up my resistance on each of my exercises.

To add muscle to your pectorals and make your chest thicker, you must get your muscles stronger. You must force your body to handle heavier and heavier resistance on all your exercises. And, of course, make certain that each exercise is done in good form.

Ray always trained that way, and so should you.

Chapter 21

UPPER ARMS:
LOADING YOUR GUNS

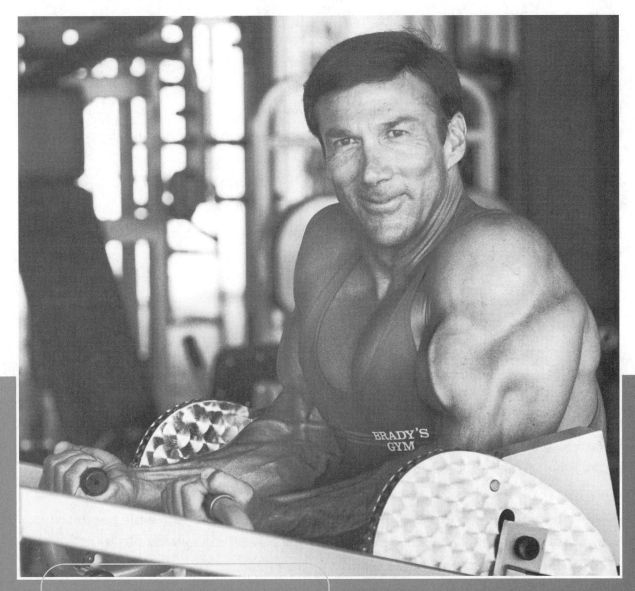

I became friends with Boyer Coe in 1965 at the Mr. Texas contest, which he easily won. This photo was taken at the Nautilus headquarters in 1983. Today, at almost 60 years of age, Coe still has award-winning biceps and triceps.

"I CAN ADD a quarter of an inch on my arms by just thinking about training them," Arthur Jones once said to me.

Almost anyone else would think Jones was kidding, but I believed him. Of course, I'd actually seen him train his arms. The level of concentration he put into every repetition was beyond belief, unless you saw it.

Most lifters will grimace and moan as if they're in a torture chamber, especially during the final reps of an all-out set. Not Jones. He never changed expression, always kept his face and neck relaxed, and never even shifted his gaze. You wouldn't know he was working to full capacity until afterward, when you'd see the size of his pumped-up arm muscles. (And, of course, there were the long-term results of his efforts, which were equally obvious.)

"When I really focus on doing a curl," Jones said, "muscular contractions begin occurring in my biceps before overt movement is noted. Thus, after laying off from training for several months, the mere thought of working my arms produces an overnight increase in their size."

Exercise physiologists have found a basis for Jones's belief that his mind could build muscle. When they placed a device called an electromyograph on certain muscle groups and instructed study subjects to think about contracting the muscles without actually doing so, they detected tiny signals of activity in those tissues. Their muscles, for lack of a better word, were rehearsing the actual movement that was occurring only in the study subjects' brains.

Mind over Muscle

Most lifters look at the muscle-building process as something that's almost entirely physical. But mental practice—seeing a performance in your imagination—is also important.

Jones wasn't the only one who used his brain to build his biceps. Boyer Coe, whom I trained many times in 1983, seemed to think about each repetition as he applied slow, deliberate form throughout his workouts. Besides being 1969 Mr. America, Coe won the Mr. Universe title four times, the Mr. World title five times, and dozens of Best Arms awards.

The primary advantage of this type of practice is that you can mentally perform your workouts using proper form and intensity, making repetition increases in all your exercises, 100 percent of the time. You'll never have a bad workout, and you'll always accomplish your goal—given that you know how to achieve your objective. Such preparation can definitely be a boon to building big arms.

So establish your goal, plan your attack, and focus precisely with both physical and mental assaults.

HIT Arm Cycles

Because arms are such a popular body part to work, I'm going to present three somewhat different routines, all of which involve variations of the biceps curl, triceps extension, chinup, and dip. The first routine provides an interesting take on reverse pre-exhaustion. The second routine involves normal pre-exhaustion, and the third routine pushes double pre-exhaustion.

Primary Function of the Biceps

The primary function of the biceps is supination, or twisting of the hand. On the right arm, the biceps supinates the hand in a clockwise direction; on the left, the twisting is done counterclockwise. The bending action accomplished by the biceps is strictly secondary.

One simple test will prove this: Bend your forearm toward your upper arm as far as possible, while keeping your hand pronated (palm down). Place your other hand on the biceps of the bent arm. Note that your biceps is not contracted, even though the bending action has been completed. In other words, though your arm is bent as far as possible, your biceps has performed only part of its function. Now twist the hand on your bent arm into a supinated position and feel your biceps contract. Full contraction of the biceps results in twisting your hand and forearm, and your biceps cannot fully contract unless the twisting occurs.

For this reason, you can curl more with your palms turned up than you can with a reverse-curl grip, in which your palms are down. Your biceps are prevented from twisting into full contraction in the reverse-curl position, which means that it's impossible to involve all the available muscle fibers in the exercise.

Another important point: You won't get as good a workout when you do biceps work with an easy-curl bar, which moves your hands toward pronation and away from supination. It does not fully pronate your hands, but it goes too far to permit your biceps to function best.

That's why any exercise for the biceps should be done with a fully supinated, palms-up grip.

Reverse Pre-Exhaustion Cycle

1. Extremely slow chinup, 1 repetition only, immediately followed by

2. Biceps curl with barbell

3. Extremely slow dip, 1 repetition only, immediately followed by

4. Triceps extension with one dumbbell

Extremely slow chinup: The objective is to make a single repetition as intense and slow as possible, while still being able to complete it. From a hanging, underhand position with arms straight, take as long as possible to get your chin over the bar. Try to move an inch and hold, another inch and hold, and so on. Remain in each position briefly (without lowering) and move up very deliberately until your chin is over and your upper chest touches the bar. Have an assistant who has a watch with a second hand call out your time in seconds (5, 10, 15, 20) as the exercise progresses. Once you've achieved the top position, lower yourself in exactly the same manner. Again, your assistant should call out your time in seconds. Begin this movement with a goal of 30 seconds positive (pulling yourself up) and 30 seconds negative (lowering). If successful, add 5 seconds to both phases. *Note:* Only a handful of bodybuilders have ever been able to achieve 60 seconds up and 60 seconds down. At the completion of the slow descent, move quickly to the biceps curl.

Biceps curl with barbell: To be conservative, lower your normal curling resistance by at least 20 percent. Pick up the barbell with your palms up and your hands shoulder width apart. Stand erect.

Just how big is a 20-inch arm? I accurately measured the height of Eddie Robinson's flexed arm, as determined by a caliper, at 7³/₈ inches. Then I taped the circumference of his arm at barely under 20¹/₂ inches. Robinson's arm on this page is exactly 7³/₈ inches thick, or life-size.

While keeping your body straight, smoothly curl the barbell. Slowly lower while keeping your elbows stable. Do not pause at the bottom. Begin the next repetition immediately. Repeat for maximum repetitions. Focus on getting 1 more repetition, even when it looks as if you won't succeed. Make it. Get a quick drink of water and ready yourself for the extremely slow dip.

Extremely slow dip: The 1-repetition dip is performed in a similar fashion to the 1-repetition chinup. Start the dip in the bottom, stretched position. Take 30 to 60 seconds to push to the top and an equal amount of time to lower. Your training partner should make sure that he paces you appropriately by calling out your raising and lowering times in seconds. After the last few seconds of lowering, step down, pick up a properly loaded dumbbell, and start doing the triceps extension.

Triceps extension with one dumbbell: Grab a single dumbbell at one end with both hands and press it overhead. Be sure to keep your elbows close to your ears as you lower the dumbbell slowly behind your head. Keep your upper arms vertical; only your forearms and hands should move. Extend the dumbbell smoothly back to the top position. Repeat until you reach muscular failure.

Normal Pre-Exhaustion Cycle

1. Biceps curl with barbell, immediately followed by

2. Chinup, negative only

3. Triceps extension with one dumbbell, immediately followed by

4. Dip, negative only

Biceps curl with barbell: Give the curl your entire focus as you grind out a strict 8 to 12 repetitions. Afterward, immediately head over to the chinning bar.

Chinup, negative only: If you can attach some additional resistance around your waist and do at least 6 negative repetitions, do it. If not, stick with only your body weight. Either way, climb fast and lower slowly. Make sure, also, that you lower all the way to the bottom, stretched position. Don't shorten the range. Get as many repetitions as you can before you lose control. Rest a minute, get a drink, and prepare for the triceps extension.

Triceps extension with one dumbbell: Extend the dumbbell smoothly and lower it slowly for 8 to 12 strict repetitions. After you get the last possible repetition, go to the dip bars.

Dip, negative only: Climb quickly and lower yourself slowly—with or without added resistance—for 8 to 12 repetitions. Dig deep and hold your form as best you can. It really helps to think about relaxing your face and neck on each repetition.

Double Pre-Exhaustion Cycle

You'd better have your act together to progress through this cycle. It's for the well-conditioned, advanced bodybuilder only.

1. Extremely slow chinup, 1 repetition only, immediately followed by

2. Biceps curl with barbell, immediately followed by

3. Chinup, negative only

4. Extremely slow dip, 1 repetition only, immediately followed by

5. Triceps extension with one dumbbell, immediately followed by

6. Dip, negative only

Extremely slow chinup, 1 repetition only: If you haven't done this exercise before, try 30 seconds up and 30 seconds down. You're in for a treat. Make sure you spend as much time on the negative as you do on the positive. It helps to have a training partner call out your time in seconds.

Biceps curl with barbell: Start curling immediately. Keep the repetitions as strict as possible and go until failure.

Chinup, negative only: This is a real test for your biceps strength: Can you do an 8-second repetition with 40 pounds attached to your waist? How about a second repetition, then a third? Eight repetitions is your goal, with or without the added resistance. (You can also use a combination of both—as many reps as you can manage with the weighted belt, then a few more with just your body weight.) Shake your arms a bit, wash your mouth out, and jump back into the cycle.

Extremely slow dip, 1 repetition only: Just like the slow chinup, try to take at least 30 seconds going to the top position and the same amount of time fighting your way down.

Triceps extension with one dumbbell: Grab a dumbbell at one end with both hands and let your triceps do their thing. Burn 'em out, brother.

Dip, negative only: Mount the dip bars, preferably with some resistance attached to a weight belt, and begin the deliberate lowering process. Make up your mind that your somewhat rested chest and shoulder muscles can be called into action to make your triceps simply do more work—more work than they've done previously. Now make it happen for 8 or more good repetitions.

An Interesting Twist

My favorite HIT arm routine is the first one, the reverse pre-exhaustion cycle. Here's something you can try on the chinup and the dip. Instead of starting with 30 seconds positive and 30 seconds negative, begin with the negative, then the positive, and end with another negative. So you're actually doing 1½ repetitions as follows: 30 seconds negative, 30 seconds positive, and 30 seconds negative. You are doubling up on the negative, which makes the exercise harder.

All three of the arm cycles emphasize negative work, which is a surefire way to kick-start your biceps and triceps to growth.

After the Arm Cycle

To complete your routine, all you need are four or two exercises, depending on the specific arm cycle you select. I suggest the leg press, the seated calf raise, and the front flexion and back extension on the four-way neck machine. For a two-exercise addition, simply drop the neck exercises.

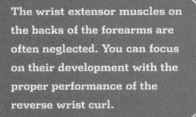

Chapter 22

FOREARMS:
BUNDLES OF STEEL CABLES

The wrist extensor muscles on the backs of the forearms are often neglected. You can focus on their development with the proper performance of the reverse wrist curl.

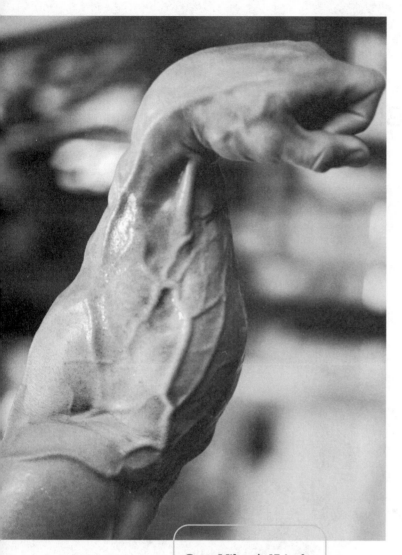

Scott Wilson's 15-inch forearm appears to be composed of steel cables.

WHEN I MET Scott Wilson at the Orlando International Airport in 1984, I did a double take on his forearms. He was wearing a blue sweatshirt with the sleeves cut off at the elbows, and he was carrying two good-sized bags in each hand. You couldn't help noticing the huge, tan forearms that looked as if they had been assembled with bunches of steel cables. I still think those were the leanest, most defined forearms I've ever seen.

He had just competed in a professional contest in Toronto, and I offered to help him with his bags. I picked one up, and it must've weighed at least 30 pounds.

But he declined my offer, saying he had all the bags arranged for balance; removing one would make it more difficult to walk with the other three. (Later, I found out that he always carried a pair of adjustable dumbbells with him to competitions, along with 50 pounds of weight plates distributed evenly among the four bags.)

When I marveled at the size, definition, and vascularity of Wilson's forearms to Chris Lund, who'd traveled with him from Toronto, Lund noted that Wilson's forearms had been the object of scrutiny throughout the trip. "One guy even accused him of smuggling heroin in his forearms."

"Well, if that guy's right," I said, "then Scott's forearms must be worth a million dollars."

Million-Dollar Forearms

A forearm, according to Arthur Jones, is properly measured cold with a thin-paper tape, with the elbow straight and the wrist flexed. The tape goes snuggly around the largest part of the forearm, and the measurement is taken to the nearest $1/16$ inch.

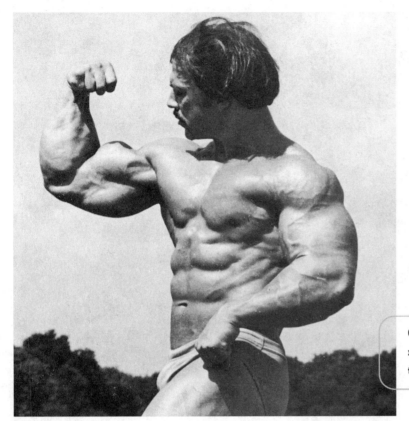

Casey Viator's 15⁷/₁₆-inch right forearm is shown to advantage here.

Here are some of Jones's largest measurements.

- Franco Columbu: 13¼ inches

- Bill Pearl: 13¾ inches

- Arnold Schwarzenegger: 13¹⁵/₁₆ inches

- Boyer Coe: 14 inches

- Scott Wilson: 15 inches

- Mike Mentzer: 15¼ inches

- Casey Viator: 15⁷/₁₆ inches

- Sergio Oliva: 15⁹/₁₆ inches

- Ray Mentzer: 15⁹/₁₆ inches

Oliva weighed 233 pounds at the time of the measurement, and he was in top shape. Ray Mentzer weighed 260, but he wasn't. But the most impressive of those measurements, in my opinion, was Vi-ator's 15⁷/₁₆-inch forearms, at a body weight of 218 pounds. (The largest forearm measurement I know of was Bill Kazmaier, once known as the world's strongest man. In his prime, Kazmaier's forearm measured 17½ inches, which in Arthur Jones's strict style would be approximately 16¾ inches. He weighed 340 pounds at a height of 6 feet 4 inches.)

But for pure visual appeal, Wilson had the best forearms I've ever seen. You'd need his genetics to build a pair of forearms like his—including long muscle bellies in the lower arms—but anyone can improve dramatically on what they have now.

HIT Forearm Cycle

The biggest problem with forearm training is the short range of motion. That's why you need to

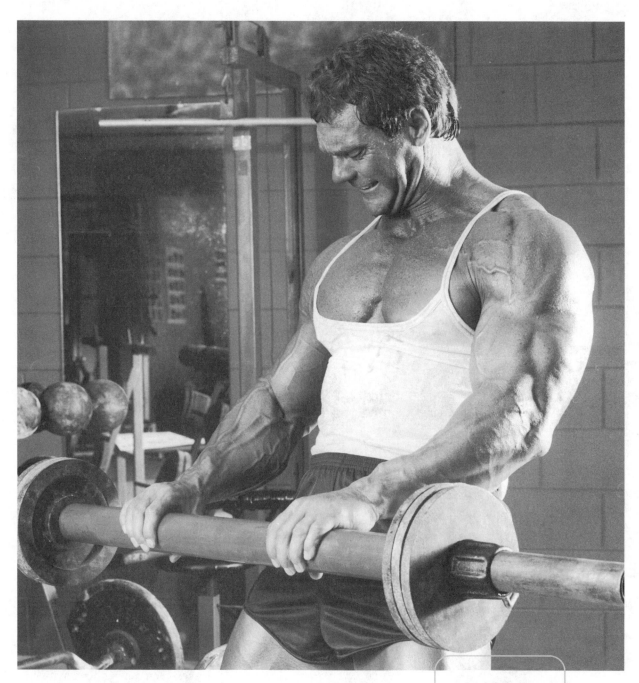

A thick-handled barbell adds an interesting variation to your forearm routine. If one is available, try it for the reverse curl.

do four exercises in a row for complete stimulation in those muscles. If you have access to a thick-handled barbell, experiment with it on some of the exercises. It definitely brings a different feel to the hands and forearms. Let's examine the sequence.

1. Wrist curl with barbell, immediately followed by

2. Finger curl with barbell, immediately followed by

3. Reverse wrist curl with barbell, immediately followed by

4. Reverse curl with barbell

Wrist curl with barbell: Grasp a barbell with a palms-up grip. Rest your forearms on your thighs and the back of your hands against your knees, and sit down. Lean forward until the angle between your upper arms and forearms is 90 degrees. This allows you to isolate your forearms more completely. Curl your hands smoothly and contract your forearm flexor muscles. Pause, and then lower the barbell slowly. Repeat for maximum repetitions. Reduce the weight 25 percent and immediately start the finger curl.

Finger curl with barbell: Assume the same position as the wrist curl. Instead of moving your hands and flexing your wrists, extend your fingers. Curl the bar back to your hands with your fin-gers and repeat for 8 to 12 repetitions. Place the barbell on the floor, lighten the resistance, and do the reverse wrist curl.

Reverse wrist curl with barbell: Assume the same position as for the wrist curl, except reverse your grip. Move the backs of your hands upward and extend your wrists. Pause in the top position. Lower slowly to the stretched position. Repeat for maximum repetitions. Move quickly to a heavier barbell for the reverse curl.

Reverse curl with barbell: This exercise will finish off your fatigued forearms. Grasp a barbell with a palms-down grip and stand. Stabilize your elbows against your sides and keep them there throughout the exercise. Curl the barbell. Lower slowly to the bottom. Repeat for 8 to 12 repetitions.

Forearm Forging

Instead of working your targeted muscles first, which I recommend in most of the specialized routines, I want you to do the other four exercises in the workout first and hit your forearms last. For example, you could do the leg curl, leg press, bent-over row, and incline bench press. Then, forge your forearms with the four-exercise cycle.

You'll be glad you did, especially if you ever find yourself carrying 50 pounds of dumbbells through an airport.

Chapter 23

WAIST:
ETCHING A SIX-PACK

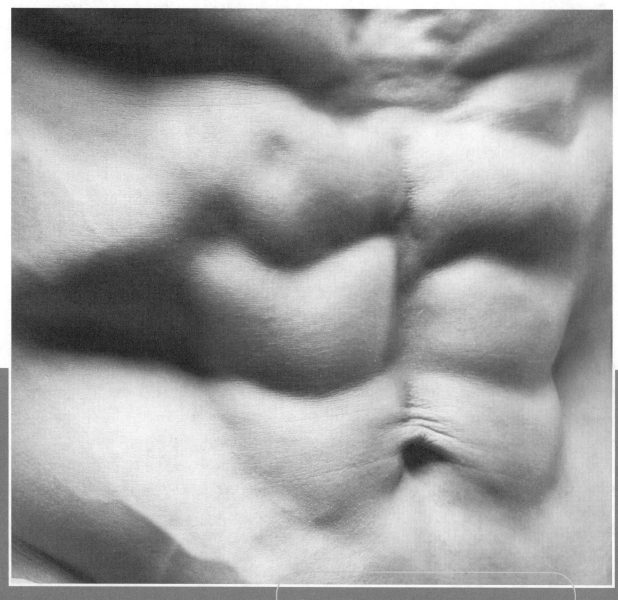

That sought-after six-pack formation shows clearly on the midsection of Andy McCutcheon, who demonstrates the HIT exercises throughout this book.

WHEN I BEGAN bodybuilding in the early 1960s, nobody thought much about lean waistlines or ripped abdominals. We were into building big arms and pecs, broad shoulders, flared lats, and muscular calves. We wanted to gain weight—or bulk, as we called it back then. I know I just wanted to weigh 200 pounds.

Of course, I had an ulterior motive for bulking up. I had played quarterback and middle linebacker at Conroe High School, and one of my goals was to play football at Baylor University in Waco, Texas. I figured that the bigger and stronger I was, the better my chance of making the team. I was right. I entered Baylor at 208 pounds, made the team, and started in two of the five freshman games in 1962. The problem was that I had to play offensive tackle instead of my customary skill positions. I would've been a big quarterback at 208, but instead I was a small left tackle.

One season in the trenches was enough. Instead of playing football in 1963, I decided to concentrate on strength training and bodybuilding at the local gym in Waco. The gym's owner, Ed Cook, had placed second to John Gourgott in the 1960 Southern USA contest.

And, more to the point of this chapter, Cook had the best abdominals I'd ever seen at that time.

More Than a Ripple

Ed Cook was about 5 feet 8 inches tall and weighed 175 pounds—not that big but very muscular, especially throughout his torso. He could pop out each row of his abdominal muscles, starting at the top and working down. He seemed to have paper-thin skin on his torso and arms, which won him a lot of physique shows.

I trained at Cook's gym for 3 years and eventually got to the point where I could match or beat him on all muscle groups except abdominals.

Cook used a standard split routine: 2 days per week upper body, and 2 days per week lower body. But each of his four weekly workouts began the same way: three high-repetition sets of bent-knee situps, alternated with three high-repetition sets of leg raises. He'd do as many as 50 reps per set, and if he was preparing for a contest, he repeated the routine at the end of each workout.

Lots of bodybuilders, like Cook, believed that abdominals required that kind of volume and frequency. And, in Cook's case, it was hard to argue with the results. Me? I struggled for 10 years to figure out the science behind building a six-pack and then stripping off enough fat to make it show.

Into the Gene Pool

Your personal genetics limit what you can and cannot do in life. As I explained in chapter 7, to achieve a really big arm, you have to have long muscle bellies and short tendons in your biceps and your triceps. Many guys who get interested in bodybuilding quickly lose interest when they figure out that, no matter what they do, they'll never develop exceptionally big arms.

On the other hand, the rare guy who does have exceptional length in his biceps and triceps achieves great results from just lifting the phone to his ear.

I believe that genetics affect your ab development in three ways.

Low level of body fat. It's possible to have great abdominals that go unnoticed—if they're covered by fat. The average man in the United States has a body that's about 25 percent fat. The average bodybuilder entering a physique contest today has about 12 percent body fat. The ones who win the top prizes, however, have less than 5 percent. And the guys with the ripped abs, the ones who look as though all the fat has been surgically removed from their midsections, will be at the 3 percent level.

Fat on your body is stored in microscopically small cells that have the capacity to swell or shrink. Gain fat, and they swell; lose fat, and they shrink. More important, however, is the fact that the total number of fat cells in your body is inherited and subject to a huge variation based on your ancestors' fatness or leanness. The leanest guy you see on a fitness-equipment infomercial will probably still have at least 10 billion fat cells, but someone who's morbidly obese might have 250 billion. You're probably somewhere in the middle of those extremes, and that means you can't get down to 5 percent body fat no matter how hard you try. Unless you're one of the lucky few with 10 to 12 billion fat cells, it can't possibly happen.

And how do you know if you're in that range? You could undergo multiple fat biopsies throughout your body, then have the samples counted using an electron microscope. That would be very time consuming, not to mention expensive. Or you could do a simple self-test.

Because 50 percent of your fat is located directly under your skin, pinch a double layer of skin and fat at various spots on and around your midsection.

Notice how thick that double layer is. Now do the same pinch on the back of your hand, where you have very few fat cells. Guys with a low number of fat cells will have skin that's about equally thick in both places, usually $1/8$ inch or less. But if you're more typical and have, say, a $1/2$-inch or $3/4$-inch pinch on your midsection, you have considerably more fat cells.

Favorable ordering of spots from which you lose fat. Your body has a genetically determined pattern for storing fat and an inverse pattern for losing it. A typical guy deposits fat first on the sides of his waist—in his love handles. Second, it goes over the navel area, then to the hips and chest, the upper arms and thighs, and finally the calves, forearms, hands, feet, and head. When he reduces fat, it comes off in reverse order: first from the head, feet, hands, forearms, and calves; then from the thighs and upper arms, followed by the chest and hips, and finally the navel area and sides.

But a few people have different fat-storage patterns. These people lose fat first or second from their midsections. Where you and I struggle to lose an inch from our waists, they do it easily.

Symmetrically paired abdominal muscles. Most people who are extremely lean in the midsection can display three paired rectangular blocks of muscle. You know this as the six-pack, of course. (Some very lucky people have a fourth pair of blocks.) These blocks are caused by strips of tendons, the thickest of which runs vertically down the middle. Three or four other tendons run horizontally and connect to the vertical tendon on both sides.

Many times, the left muscle blocks don't match

the blocks on the right. Sometimes the right muscle is thicker than the left. Or the tendons on the left side aren't parallel to the ones on the right. Or perhaps the tendons are wavy instead of straight. In a bodybuilding contest, the judges usually prefer the symmetrical, evenly developed blocks with parallel tendons.

So the look most guys want, the symmetrical six-pack, is also genetic—not to mention rare.

The Paradox

When someone has both great genetics and a perfect six-pack, he could have gotten that six-pack in any number of ways. He could have terrific abdominals in spite of his training, not because of it. (Although if you ask him, he'll almost certainly believe that his diet and exercise plan produced the abs that were in his genetic code all along.) On the other hand, people with average genetics—about 80 percent of the population—have to work very hard to get into decent shape. And after years and years of training, they still won't have the same level of abdominal sharpness as people with exceptional genetics who don't work nearly as hard.

When I look back on my training experience with Ed Cook, I realize that Ed had all the genetic requirements for great abs. He had a low level of body fat and very thin skin, the ability to lose fat initially from his midsection, and symmetrically paired abdominal muscles. Did he understand proper training for his midsection? Ed was a nice guy, and I learned a great deal from him, but no, he didn't understand how to train the abdominals.

It's been proven *repeatedly* that spot reduction of fat around your waist isn't possible through high-repetition situps, leg raises, side bends, or any other exercise.

So be realistic. Don't expect to get a deeply etched six-pack formation unless you already have a pretty good one. If you can't tell, get lean first by reducing your dietary calories, then reevaluate.

Regardless, you can still strengthen your midsection muscles significantly by practicing a HIT routine that emphasizes an abdominal cycle. The following routine does just that.

HIT Midsection Cycle

1. Side bend with one dumbbell, immediately followed by

2. Reverse trunk curl on floor, immediately followed by

3. Trunk curl on floor, immediately followed by

4. Chinup, negative only

Side bend with one dumbbell: Grasp a heavy dumbbell in your right hand. Stand erect and place your left hand on top of your head. Bend to your right. This bending stretches your left obliques. Return smoothly to the erect position. Repeat the bending to your right side for 8 to 12 repetitions. Switch the dumbbell to your left hand, place your right hand on top of your head, and perform an equal number of side bends to your left side.

Reverse trunk curl on floor: This is a terrific exercise, especially if you've never tried it correctly. Lie faceup on the floor with your hands on both sides of your hips. Bring your thighs to your chest, so that your knees and hips are in a flexed position,

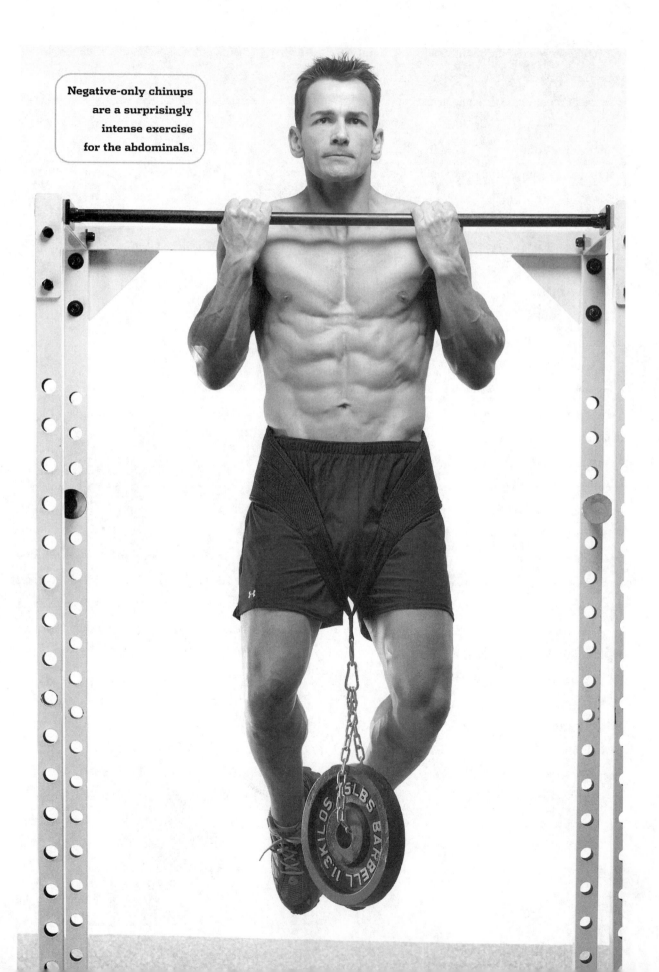

Negative-only chinups are a surprisingly intense exercise for the abdominals.

and cross your lower legs at your ankles. Curl your pelvic area toward your chest by lifting your buttocks and lower back. Pause in the contracted position. Lower your buttocks slowly to the floor. Try not to move your knees and lower legs. Keep them near your chest throughout the lifting and lowering. Repeat for 8 to 12 repetitions.

Trunk curl on floor: This exercise activates your rectus abdominis (the six-pack muscle) by relaxing your iliopsoas muscles (commonly called the hip flexors). Lie faceup on the floor and bring your heels up close to your buttocks. Put the soles of your feet together and spread your knees wide. Widen your elbows and cup your hands around your ears. Doing so prevents unnecessary pulling on your head. Focus on curling your head, shoulders, and upper back off the floor ever so slowly. Pause when you can't go any higher (the range of motion is very short). Pull with your abdominal muscles, not your hands or shoulders. Lower your upper back and shoulders to the floor. Repeat for 8 to 12 repetitions. When you can do more than 12 repetitions, hold a 10-pound weight plate across your upper chest.

Chinup, negative only: This exercise, performed immediately after the other three, will add the final touch to your abdominals. Use a Nautilus multi-exercise machine for the chin, if it's available. Grasp the crossbar with an underhand grip. Climb the steps until your chin is above the crossbar. Remove your feet from the steps, bend your knees, and lower your body slowly, inch by inch, to a full hanging position. When you get halfway down, look up, arch your lower back, and force your knees backward. Try to stretch your body completely in the bottom position before you make contact with the floor. Climb back quickly to the top position and repeat for maximum repetitions. When the exercise becomes easier, add weight to your waist with the padded belt.

Other Exercises

Your other four exercises might be as follows: leg press, stiff-legged deadlift, overhead press, and bent-arm fly. Perform them first, then do the abdominal cycle.

Finishing Touches

Don't make the mistake of training your midsection more frequently or with higher repetitions than your other muscles. Remember, spot reduction of fat isn't possible.

If you have too much fat around your waistline, then you probably have too much fat over the rest of your body as well. Adhere to a lower-calorie eating plan, which I'll cover in part V, to reduce your body fat, and train your entire body in the prescribed HIT fashion.

Part V describes how one bodybuilder turned his entire thinking and training upside-down to achieve his goals of losing fat and building muscle in the most efficient manner.

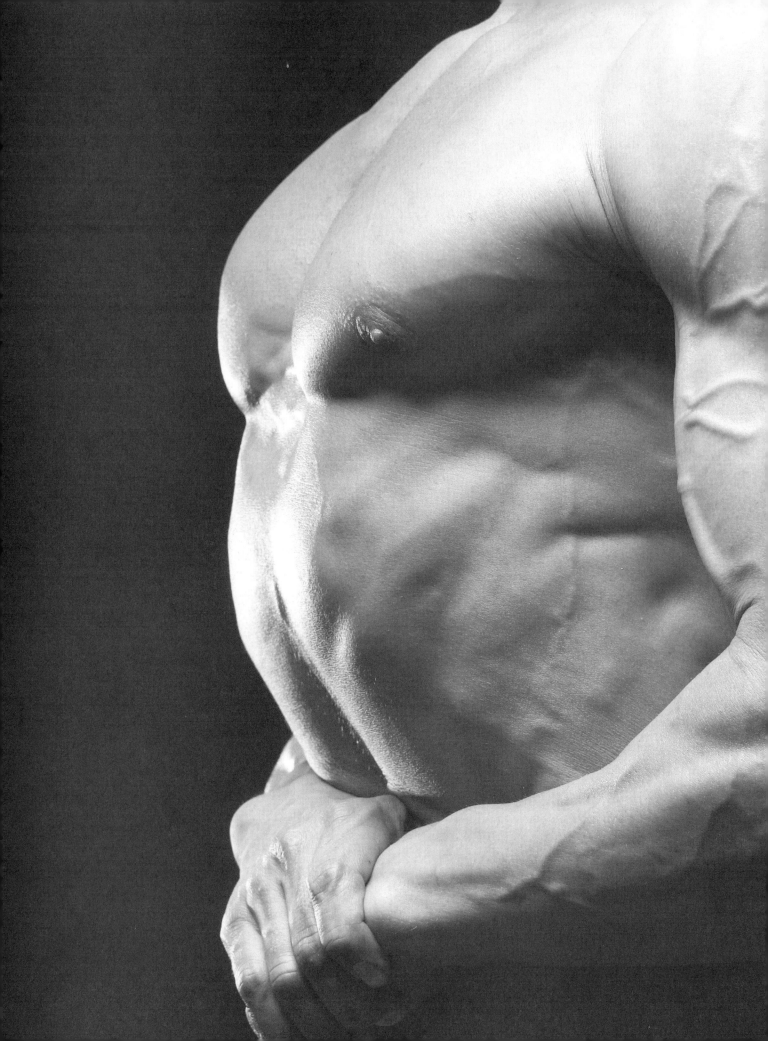

BODY TRANSFORMATION: A 6-MONTH HIT COURSE FOR EXPLOSIVE GROWTH

The next five chapters provide
a step-by-step HIT course to
transform your physique in
6 months or less.

Chapter 24

"DO THE OPPOSITE!": TURNING BODYBUILDING RIGHT SIDE UP

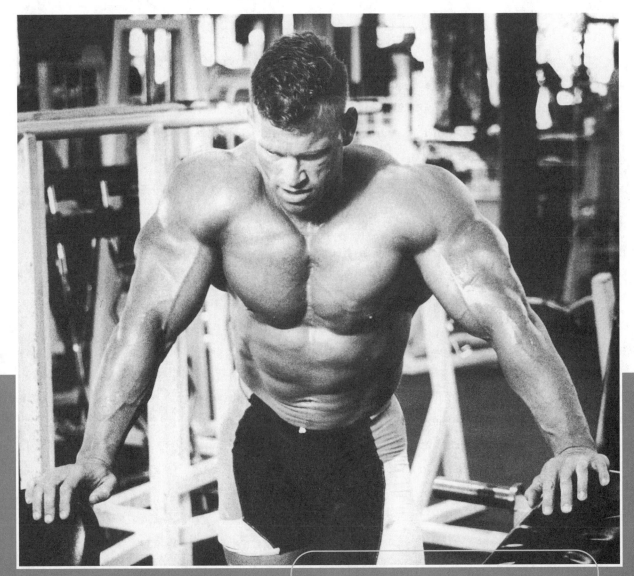

Don't be afraid to turn your back on what you see being practiced in most gyms. Keith Whitley did just that in 1990, when he switched from high volume to HIT. Whitley was rewarded when he gained 29 pounds of muscle in 42 days.

ARTHUR JONES HAD an intriguing take on the ideal workout and diet plan: "If you want to know the truth about exercising and eating, prepare a list of the most relevant questions. Now, ask these questions to a bodybuilder—the biggest, strongest bodybuilder you can find.

"Make note of the bodybuilder's answers—then do exactly the opposite.

"If he says right, go left. If he points down, climb up. If he mentions fast, move slow. At the very least, applying the opposite for each of his answers will be closer to the truth than will be his original responses."

As I'm sure you've noticed by now, Jones is an entertaining storyteller. When Jones would make his pronouncement about doing the opposite of bodybuilders, fitness-minded people in his audiences always enjoyed a good laugh. The bodybuilders in attendance, however, didn't react that way. They'd usually sit quietly for a moment, digesting what they'd heard, then tighten their lips and shake their heads.

But some bodybuilders realized that Jones was right. A few even reached out and tried to learn what Jones was willing to teach. I was one of those bodybuilders in 1970. In part I, I chronicled some of my experiences with Jones, which eventually led to my researching and writing dozens of books about high-intensity training.

But no matter how much I wrote, my message was diluted by the array of books, articles, and videotapes that preached the contrary. As I said earlier in this book, the propaganda is worse today than it was two decades ago, simply because there are more magazines and Web sites feeding a popu-lation that is more interested in the subject of building muscle.

I see thousands of bodybuilders in my travels who are upset because they aren't getting the development they had expected from their training. When confused, they naturally look to bigger, more advanced bodybuilders for advice.

Each time I observe this, I'm reminded of Arthur Jones's do-the-opposite philosophy. It was with that in mind that I teamed up with a buddy in Gainesville, Florida.

But first, a little background is necessary.

Time for Change

In 1986, Jones sold Nautilus to a group in Dallas, Texas. Being originally from Texas, I decided to join the new company in Dallas. Jones started another business, called MedX, which focused on computerized lumbar-spine strength testing. His new operation was located in Ocala, Florida, which was 60 miles west of Lake Helen. Ocala was also near the University of Florida in Gainesville, where Jones planned to do research with his lumbar-spine machine.

The new Nautilus management group in Dallas struggled for several years. Nautilus was sold again—twice, in fact. By 1990, I'd had enough and moved back to Florida. I settled in Gainesville, where Joe Cirulli had the largest, best-equipped fitness center I'd ever seen anywhere. I'd supervised several major fat-loss studies in 1985 at Cirulli's club, so I knew that the Gainesville Health and Fitness Center would be an ideal location to continue my research and writing.

That's where I met David Hudlow. Hudlow grew

up in Georgia, started strength training and body-building when he was in high school, played football for a while at Georgia Tech, was in the U.S. Marine Corps for 3 years, and ended up at the University of Florida, where he was majoring in chemistry. At the fitness center, he had a part-time job as a supervisor in the strength-training area.

He was familiar with Jones's writings and my books. As a result, I frequently asked him to help with the tests and measurements of the people participating in my exercise and diet studies. He was precise and reliable, traits that weren't easy to find among the 100 or more instructors at the fitness center.

As Hudlow and I became better friends, I could tell he was frustrated by his own personal training. In fact, like many bodybuilders I had been associated with in the past, he had reached a plateau and was baffled as to what to do. I invited him to attend the next Arthur Jones/MedX seminar, which was held the following Friday near the campus.

Jones began his presentation with his do-the-opposite story, and Hudlow found himself inspired to train hard again. Hudlow and I decided, over lunch, that we'd turn his motivation into a multiple-month experiment to document exactly what was happening to his body. In time, we started referring to the project as "upside-down bodybuilding."

We hoped for some impressive results to show that we were on the right side.

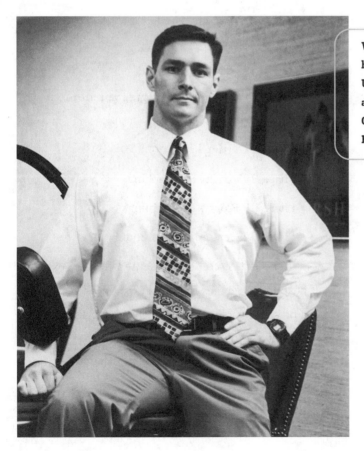

When I met David Hudlow, he was a student at the University of Florida and a supervisor at the Gainesville Health and Fitness Center.

Negative Exercise and Soreness

Negative exercise, if you aren't used to it, will make you very sore. The soreness results from several factors.

First, negative exercise involves more muscle fibers. Second, because of the greater number of muscle fibers, a deeper inroad into your starting level of strength is possible. Third, negative exercise provides more stretching to your muscles and connective tissues.

You feel negative-induced soreness sooner than you feel normal, positive-negative soreness. Not only does it occur sooner, but it goes away faster.

Don't be afraid of soreness. Simply work through it and use it as an indication that you are stimulating your muscles to grow at an accelerated rate.

More rest on your part is an absolute necessity during periods of negative exercise. It's very easy to overtrain. Try to get to bed an hour earlier than normal, especially on your workout days.

Make certain that you're eating your quota of calories each day. Drink plenty of fluids and water, because water is instrumental in the muscular growth process. It also helps prevent muscle cramps. If your muscles are prone to cramps after heavy negative training, you probably need to take in more fluids. It's especially important to drink 8 ounces of cold water immediately after your workout.

The Upside-Down, Right-Side-Up Challenge

Here are the popular practices we wanted to prove wrong.

- Bulking up, then getting lean

- High-protein, low-carbohydrate eating

- No emphasis on water drinking

- Long workouts

- Split routines

- Frequent, daily training

- Fast-speed repetitions

- Exhausted recovery ability

And these were our do-the-opposite alternatives.

- Getting lean, then bulking up

- High-carbohydrate, low-protein eating

- Emphasis on water drinking

- Brief workouts

- Whole-body routines

- Three-times-per-week training

- Slow-speed repetitions

- Rested recovery ability

Then, we organized our program into four segments.

- Phase I: Getting lean

- Phase II: Loading and packing

- Phase III: Progressive training

- Phase IV: Customized workouts

The entire course, presented in the next four chapters, stretches for almost 6 months. It provides a practical application of all the HIT principles.

Review the chapters carefully. They just may be your ticket to what I promise on the cover and in the introduction of this book: body transformation through explosive muscular growth.

Chapter 25

PHASE I, GETTING LEAN: A 2-WEEK QUICK START

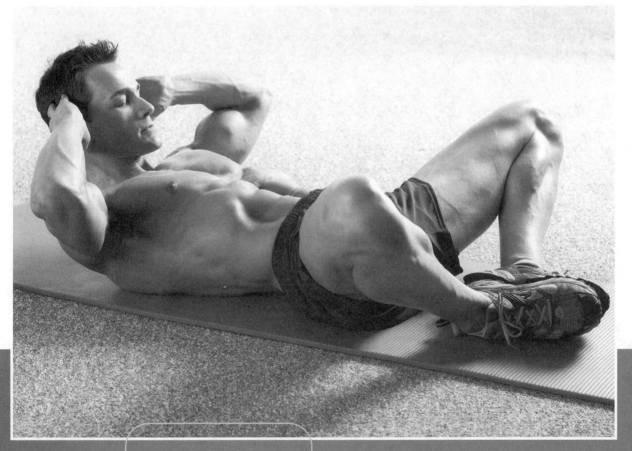

Getting lean requires a reduced-calorie eating plan combined with basic HIT exercises, such as the trunk curl for the midsection.

OUR FIRST GOAL was to get David Hudlow lean. At 27, he stood 5 feet 11½ inches, weighed 218¾ pounds, and had a 40⅝-inch waistline. His body-fat level was 28.4 percent, which meant he carried about 62 pounds of fat.

As I said in the previous chapter, most bodybuilders try to bulk up, then get lean. Hudlow was an ideal candidate for the do-the-opposite system. I wanted to reduce his body fat to 10 percent or less.

How Fat Are You Really?

Take off your shirt and look in the mirror. Place your hands behind your head and contract your abdominal muscles. Can you see clearly the three or four paired sets of muscles from top to bottom? If not, you need to get leaner.

Next, with your thumb and index finger, grasp a vertical fold of skin on the right side of your navel. Using a ruler, measure the thickness of the skinfold. If the measurement is more than ½ inch, you're too fat. It's time for you to get serious.

A Quick Start: Lose 10 Pounds in 2 Weeks

The outlined 2-week routine that follows is designed to act as a quick start, in that it may be completed prior to a more comprehensive fat-loss program. If you have more than 15 pounds of fat to lose, you need to understand that it's going to take months, not weeks, to eliminate it. You can find several long-term eating programs that are adaptable for 6 to 12 weeks in my previous book, *The Bowflex Body Plan*. For now, though, try this quick-start course, which includes three steps.

1. Eat 1,500 calories each day. The quick-start eating plan consists of three meals and two snacks per day. All the meals and snacks are carbohydrate-rich, with moderate amounts of fat and protein. Research shows that men can consume the same breakfast and lunch each day for 14 days. This simplifies the eating and can make the calorie counting more efficient. Be sure to take a multivitamin with minerals daily, one that doesn't contain any listed nutrient on the label that exceeds 100 percent of the Recommended Dietary Allowances. Calories for each food are listed in parentheses.

Breakfast = Approximately 400 Calories

1 bagel—plain, blueberry, or oat bran—Sara Lee, frozen, toasted (210)

1 ounce light cream cheese (60)

4 dried pitted prunes (80)

½ cup orange juice (55)

Noncaloric beverage

Lunch = Approximately 400 Calories

Sandwich, consisting of:

2 slices whole-grain bread (140)

1 tablespoon light mayonnaise (50)

1 tablespoon sweet pickle relish (20)

2 tomato slices (14)

4 ounces white meat chicken or turkey (160)

Noncaloric beverage

Afternoon Snack = Approximately 150 Calories

Choose one of three foods:

- 1 cup low-fat flavored yogurt (check the calorie count on the label and adjust appropriately) (150)

- Fresh fruit—such as a large banana, orange, pear, or apple (150)

Dark Eyes, Dark Skin, and Leanness

If a computer were programmed to analyze the physical characteristics of the winners of major bodybuilding championships over the last 50 years, an unexpected factor would surface: The vast majority of the winners would have dark eyes, dark hair, and dark skin. A high correlation would exist between low body fat—otherwise known as "muscle definition"—and dark skin, eyes, and hair. There would be a few light-skinned, blue-eyed, blond-haired champions (Dorian Yates being the most obvious), but they'd be the exceptions.

One explanation is the climates from which different body types emerge. A strong relationship seems to exist between body fat and annual mean temperature. The colder the mean temperature, the fatter people become. The warmer the mean temperature, the leaner they are. The relative leanness of warm-dwelling people and the relative fatness of cold-dwelling people can be traced back to a period roughly 18,000 to 25,000 years ago. Back then, in the cold regions of the world, the ability to store surplus fat under the skin with the least possible total food intake may have made the difference between life and death.

Central heating, air-conditioning, and mass production of warm clothing all serve to minimize a modern individual's exposure to environmental extremes. Even so, scientists can document the degree to which the contemporary American is still programmed by blueprints laid down by Ice Age ancestors.

What do these characteristics mean to the bodybuilder? Generally, bodybuilders with dark skin, hair, and eyes—compared with those who have light skin, blond hair, and blue eyes—have a genetic advantage that predisposes them toward lower body fat, and thus more-extreme muscular definition.

Take a good look at the fatness or leanness of your mother and father. Do the same for your grandparents. Check out the color of their eyes and hair. Now, reevaluate your body's potential for leanness—and be realistic in your assessment.

- 1 cereal-fruit snack bar—such as those made by Kellogg's, Nature Valley, Quaker, and Kashi. Check the nutritional information on the label, as carbohydrates should provide at least 50 percent of the calories, and adjust the serving size appropriately. (150)

Dinner = Approximately 400 Calories

Choice of tuna salad or one of three frozen microwave meals:

Tuna Salad Dinner

In a large bowl, mix the following:

- ½ (6-ounce) can chunk light tuna in water, drained (75)

- ½ cup (4 ounces) whole-kernel corn, canned, no salt added (60)

- ½ cup (4 ounces) dark red kidney beans, canned (65)

1 tablespoon sweet pickle relish (20)

1 tablespoon light mayonnaise (50)

2 slices whole grain bread (140)

Noncaloric beverage

Frozen Microwave Dinners

Choose one of three:

- Glazed Chicken, Lean Cuisine Everyday Favorites (230), served with 2½ slices whole grain bread (175) and a noncaloric beverage

- Blackened Chicken, Healthy Choice (320), served with 1 slice whole grain bread (70) and a noncaloric beverage

- Lasagna with Meat Sauce, Michelina's Authentico (290), served with 1½ slices whole grain bread (105) and a noncaloric beverage

Evening Snack = Approximately 150 Calories

Same as the afternoon snack.

Important Notes:

• Noncaloric beverages are any type of water, soft drink, tea, or coffee with zero calories and no caffeine.

• For whole grain bread, try to select one that lists as the first ingredient whole, sprouted, or cracked grain.

• Other frozen microwave meals may be substituted for those listed in the plan. Select one that has from 230 to 320 calories and no more than 5 to 7 grams of fat.

2. Utilize superhydration. "Superhydration" entails drinking at least 4 quarts of cold water each day. If a person doesn't consume enough water, his body will try to retain the water it does have. Kidney function is hampered, and waste products accumulate. The liver is then called on to flush out impurities. As a result, one of the liver's main functions—metabolizing stored fat into usable energy—is minimized. The traditional recommendation of eight glasses (2 quarts) per day isn't nearly enough for maximum fat loss. I recommend twice that.

Furthermore, a person can maximize calorie burn by keeping the water ice-cold. A gallon of ice-cold water (40°F) requires 123 calories of heat energy to warm it to core body temperature (98.6°F). An insulated bottle will help keep the water chilled.

3. Incorporate high-intensity exercise three times per week. More than any other component of your body over which you have control, your muscles require calories to keep warm, regulate, contract, recover, and grow. Larger, stronger muscles burn more calories, and burning more calories is a key factor in successful fat loss.

Do only one set, 3 days per week, of each of the following five exercises.

1. Leg-press machine or squat with barbell

2. Straight-arm pullover with one dumbbell

3. Bench press with barbell

4. Biceps curl with barbell

5. Trunk curl on floor

Begin with 8 repetitions and add at least 1 repetition each workout. Do as many repetitions as you can in proper form. Always work to failure. When you can do 12 or more repetitions, add resistance at your next workout.

During the initial stage of a reduced-calorie diet, it's easy to become overstressed, and a stressed system will actually preserve the fat you're trying to lose. To help with recovery, be sure to get extra rest and sleep.

Great Expectations

My research on the quick-start course shows that the average overfat bodybuilder who weighs more than 200 pounds can expect to lose 11.4 pounds of fat in the first 2 weeks. (By "overfat," I mean that his body-fat percentage is over 18 percent.) The average overfat bodybuilder under 200 pounds will

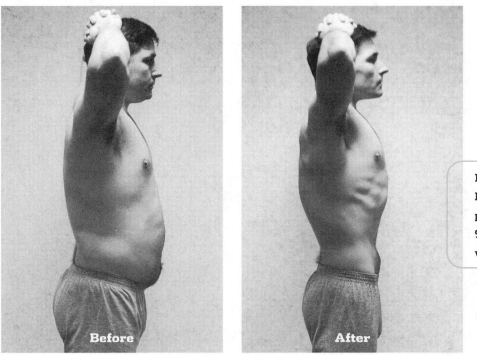

Before

After

In 66 days, David Hudlow lost 50 pounds of fat and 9¼ inches off his waist.

lose 10 to 20 percent less. Losing fat fast can definitely keep your motivation and enthusiasm at a high level as you move into the long-term program.

Hudlow adhered strictly to the 2-week course and lost 14½ pounds of fat and 3⅝ inches off his waist. He still had more adipose tissue to lose, so he shifted to one of my long-term programs (which, again, I describe in *The Bowflex Body Plan*). Fifty-two days later, he weighed 173½ pounds, having lost

50 pounds of fat and 9¼ inches off his midsection. And he built 4¾ pounds of muscle during his fat-loss process.

In 66 days, Hudlow's body fat had decreased from 28.4 to 5 percent. As a result, he was very lean when he started the loading-and-packing phase of the do-the-opposite course.

And, as you'll see in the next chapter, that worked to his advantage.

Chapter 26

PHASE II, LOADING AND PACKING: VOLUMIZING WITH CREATINE

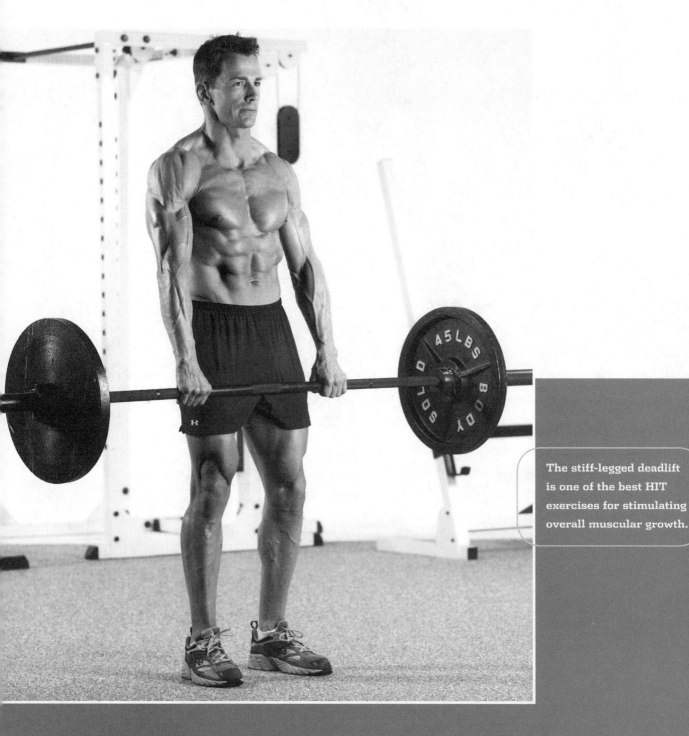

The stiff-legged deadlift is one of the best HIT exercises for stimulating overall muscular growth.

YOU'VE PROBABLY READ about, or even tried, a dietary supplement called creatine. Creatine is a proteinlike substance manufactured naturally by your body and stored in your muscles. Studies show that in your body, creatine acts the way cylinders operate in an automobile engine. When this substance is absorbed in large amounts, it's like boosting the number of cylinders in your muscles.

Over the past 10 years, thousands of so-called ergogenic aids have been introduced to the fitness scene. Once they are rigorously tested, most of these substances turn out to be nothing more than expensive placebos. Creatine, however, is one of the very few that has proven to be beneficial to the muscle-building process.

Today, at your local nutrition store, you may find all sorts of creatine products: liquid creatine, creatine with dextrose, low-carbohydrate creatine, creatine candy chews, effervescent creatine, micronized creatine, as well as plain creatine monohydrate. I've given most of these a try, but I've never had better results than with a creatine-monohydrate formula that David Hudlow and I designed for our do-the-opposite study. (Remember, Hudlow was a chemistry student at the University of Florida at the time.)

Creatine monohydrate, which is a white powder, is in theory easy to use: Mix it with water and drink. But there once were many unanswered questions: How do you get it to dissolve? What do you mix it with for maximum impact? How many times a day do you take it initially, and for how many days? (This initial part is called the "loading" phase, when you saturate your muscles with creatine. After that, you can use less and still keep your muscle levels high.)

Hudlow and I found that the best results occurred if we applied two steps. First, combine the creatine with superhydration. In other words, dissolve the daily dosage of creatine in a gallon of water and sip it continuously throughout the day. Second, add common sugar to the solution. Sugar elevates insulin levels, and insulin facilitates creatine absorption into the muscles.

Creatine-Loading Procedures

The entire process will be easier if you have these items.

1 large thermos jug, 2-gallon capacity

1 (32-ounce) plastic bottle with straw

1 battery-operated digital food scale

1 large wooden spoon

1 (5-pound) bag of granulated white sugar

1 large bottle (210 grams) of creatine monohydrate

12 ice cubes

Do the following before you begin your day.

• Pour 1 gallon of water into the jug.

• Spoon out 20, 25, or 30 grams of creatine monohydrate (1 heaping teaspoon equals approximately 5 grams, but it's best if you calculate the precise weight on the digital food scale). Use 20 grams if you weigh less than 190 pounds, 25 grams if you weigh between 190 and 220, and 30 grams if you're over 220 pounds.

• Pour the correct amount of creatine monohydrate into your water. Stir gently with the large wooden spoon for 15 seconds, or until it's dissolved.

• Weigh out 104 grams of sugar (approximately ½ cup), which has the energy value of 400 calories.

• Empty the sugar into the creatine solution and stir vigorously for 1 minute or until dissolved.

• Add ice cubes to the thermos.

• Your goal is to drink the gallon of creatine-sugar solution over the next 14 hours. Start by pouring a quart into your 32-ounce plastic bottle, and drink from that. Most people find it's easier to drink it through a straw than from a glass. Having the solution cold also helps.

• Keep refilling and drinking from your 32-ounce bottle until the thermos is empty. If possible, keep your intake consistent throughout the day, rather than drinking it all in a few hours.

• Wash the thermos and plastic bottle with hot soapy water at the end of the day.

• Repeat the same directions daily for 14 days.

• After 14 days, stop loading and move to a maintenance dosage. That's 5 grams of creatine monohydrate mixed in 4 ounces of water each morning after breakfast. Continue with the daily superhydration by drinking 1 gallon of cold water but without the sugar.

Note: Caffeine cancels some of the loading effects of creatine. Don't consume caffeinated drinks such as coffee, tea, or certain soft drinks during the loading phase.

Phase II Eating

Rather than concentrate on high-protein foods, Hudlow consumed a diet that was rich in carbohydrates and moderate in fats and proteins. He used the basic 1,500-calorie-a-day plan detailed in *The Bowflex Body Plan,* plus the 400-calorie creatine-sugar solution and 400 other calories primarily from fruit and bread. His daily totals were approximately 2,300 calories.

If you've followed the quick-start and *The Bowflex Body Plan* eating guidelines to get lean, I suggest you also raise your calories to approximately 2,300 per day for the next 2 weeks.

Phase II Exercising

For most of the time Hudlow was losing fat, he adhered to a standard HIT routine. On Monday, Wednesday, and Friday, he performed one set to failure of the following exercises: leg curl, leg extension, leg press, lateral raise, pullover, bench press, biceps curl, triceps extension, and trunk curl.

After 66 days, he took a 2-week layoff from training, then returned well-rested and enthusiastic. I revamped his schedule to include a Routine A and a Routine B for the loading-and-packing phase. He did A on Monday and Friday of the first week and on Wednesday of the second week, and B on Wednesday of the first week and Monday and Friday of the second week. (You may have seen this type of workout referred to as A-B-A, B-A-B.)

Routine A

1. Stiff-legged deadlift with barbell

2. Leg-extension machine

3. Leg-curl machine

4. Straight-arm pullover with one dumbbell

5. Biceps curl with barbell

6. Triceps pushdown on lat machine

7. Reverse curl with barbell

Routine B

1. Squat with barbell

2. Standing-calf-raise machine

3. Lateral raise with dumbbells

4. Chinup, negative only

5. Dip, negative only

6. Shoulder shrug with barbell

7. Trunk curl on floor

Massive Attack

If you've read the cover and introduction of this book, you already know that Hudlow gained 18½ pounds, all muscle, using the program listed above. His body weight increased from 173½ to 192 pounds in 14 days. His body fat stayed steady at 5 percent.

His biceps gained 1⅜ inches, his chest expanded 3 inches, and each thigh added 1⅝ inches.

Hudlow's results surpassed all my other case studies. Here's how they stack up.

Subject	Book	Muscle Pounds Gained / Weeks
Eddie Mueller	*Massive Muscles in 10 Weeks*	18¼ / 10
Eddie Mueller	*BIG*	14½ / 6*
Todd Waters	*High-Intensity Strength Training*	15¼ / 6
Jeff Turner	*Grow*	18¾ / 6
Keith Whitley	*Bigger Muscles in 42 Days*	29 / 6
David Hammond	*Bigger Muscles in 42 Days*	22½ / 6

*Yes, Mueller participated in two different projects.

As you can see, only Keith Whitley and David Hammond significantly exceeded Hudlow's results, but it took them 6 weeks to do it. The closest I've ever had to Hudlow in 2 weeks was Whitley, who gained 11¼ pounds during the initial 2-week period.

Of course, the probable world-record for muscular growth belongs to Casey Viator, who gained more than 39 pounds of muscle in 14 days during Arthur Jones's 28-day Colorado experiment. But remember, as I mentioned in chapter 3, Viator was rebuilding tissue that he had previously developed and lost due to an accident.

Personally, in my more than 35 years of training people, I've never had anyone build muscle as fast as Hudlow.

Out of curiosity, I had Hudlow's resting metabolic rate measured at the University of Florida College of Medicine, both before and after the 18½-pound muscle gain. This test is conducted following a 6-hour fast, using equipment that measures the amount of oxygen consumed and carbon dioxide expelled. At 173½ pounds, Hudlow had a resting metabolic rate of 1,552 calories per day. At 192 pounds, his rate had elevated to 2,082 calories per day. That was an increase of 530 calories, or 28.6 calories per pound of added muscle per day. In other words, each pound of muscle that Hudlow packed on his body required 28.6 calories of heat energy to keep it alive and functioning. That's proof this his added body weight was active muscle.

People Will Talk . . .

The Gainesville Health and Fitness Center is the largest facility of its kind in the United States, perhaps the world. It has more than 20,000 members, some 3,000 of whom train on an average Monday. Several hundred are hard-core bodybuilders. Be-

Results from the Loading-and-Packing Phase: 14 Days

David Hudlow's transformation was nothing short of amazing. The photos and measurements below illustrate the gains he made during phase II of the program.

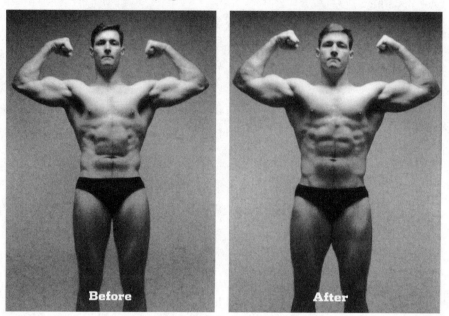

Measurement	January 11	January 25	Increase
Body weight	173½ lb	192 lb	18½ lb
Neck	15½ in	16¼ in	¾ in
Biceps*	15½ in	16⅞ in	1⅜ in
Chest	43 in	46 in	3 in
Thigh*	22⅛ in	23¾ in	1⅝ in
Calf*	14⅛ in	15⅛ in	1 in

*Note: The averaged meausurements of both arms and both legs were used in the comparisons.

cause Hudlow has been a supervisor at the club for several years, many of the bodybuilders, including the other supervisors and trainers, have been curious about his transformation. And many questioned the results, even though it all happened right before their eyes, involving someone they know.

Some suggested that the standard before-and-after photographs must have been tampered with. They were not. Others spread rumors that anabolic drugs must have been involved. Once again, they were not.

What happened is that Hudlow, in a few months, went from a pudgy fat boy to a lean, strong, muscular man.

Now, he performed negative chinups and negative dips with 90 pounds of resistance attached around his waist. He did MedX leg presses with 480 pounds on each leg. On the MedX decline bench

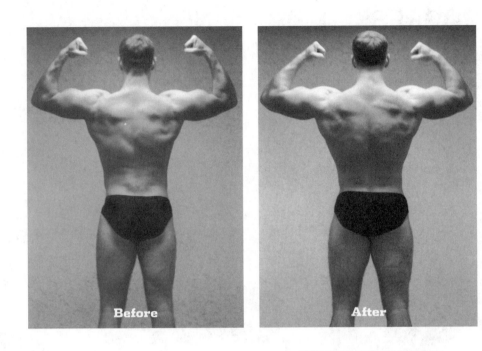

Before

After

In only 2 weeks, David Hudlow increased significantly the muscular mass of his arms, shoulders, and upper back.

press, he handled almost the entire weight stack of 500 pounds.

Of course, some people believed what they saw, and believed that Hudlow did it without drugs. Those people are asking the right questions, and some have volunteered to be subjects in my future research.

But Hudlow's gains weren't the end of the story. Phase III and phase IV were just around the corner.

Chapter 27

PHASE III, PROGRESSIVE TRAINING: ADDING CALORIES AND A LITTLE SUPERSLOW

The leg extension is an exercise that's easy to cheat on. It's to your benefit to practice the small actions that make the movement harder and thus more productive.

DAVID HUDLOW'S PROGRESSIVE-training phase included three 2-week segments, each with a unique emphasis.

- Weeks 1 and 2: Focusing on perfect form
- Weeks 3 and 4: Hitting smaller muscles
- Weeks 5 and 6: Using negative only

We also tweaked Hudlow's eating plan to give him more calories. We knew that each of the 18½ pounds of muscle he gained required an extra 25 to 30 calories per day, so we added 500 calories to the 2,300 he ate during that period. Then we added 100 more every 2 weeks. Here's how it worked.

- Weeks 1 and 2: 2,800 calories per day
- Weeks 3 and 4: 2,900 calories per day
- Weeks 5 and 6: 3,000 calories per day

Hudlow also continued using creatine monohydrate, except he stopped loading and he moved to a maintenance schedule. He took 5 grams (1 heaping teaspoon) of creatine mixed in 4 ounces of water each morning after breakfast. He no longer added sugar to the solution, but he did continue the superhydration routine of drinking at least a gallon of water each day.

Weeks 1 and 2: Focusing on Perfect Form

One of the basic principles of the do-the-opposite philosophy is the practice of slow-speed repetitions instead of fast-speed repetitions. Too many bodybuilders allow excessive momentum to pollute their sets. They start each repetition with a jerk and end each with a drop and a bang. As a result, they involve only a small portion of the targeted muscle and further subject the muscle to dangerous impact forces.

A good way to focus on perfect form is to apply SuperSlow repetitions to each exercise. SuperSlow means to lift the resistance in 10 seconds and to lower it in 10 seconds. Each repetition takes 20 seconds, which includes a smooth turnaround at both the top and the bottom.

Important: For the first workout or two, reduce your weights by 30 percent. (This is especially important if you've never tried SuperSlow.) Then increase back to your normal resistance. The idea, once you learn the form, is to move a heavy weight slowly, not a light weight slowly.

Always initiate each movement smoothly. Keep the motion steady. Do 4 to 6 repetitions. When you can do 6 perfect repetitions, increase the resistance by 2 to 3 percent at your next workout. Also note that, beginning now, your Wednesday workout of both weeks is performed not to failure (NTF), which means you must stop the set 1 repetition short of failure. Your recovery ability will get a little boost, which is good.

Here's the SuperSlow routine for weeks 1 and 2.

Perfect-Form Routine

1. Leg-curl machine

2. Leg-extension machine

3. Leg-press machine

4. Bench press with barbell

5. Shoulder shrug with barbell

6. Biceps curl with barbell

7. Regular chinup/Regular dip (alternate them)

Remember, you'll be training on a Monday-Wednesday-Friday schedule, but your Wednesday workout will be not to failure (NTF).

Cats Build Muscle

When I was in Dallas in the late 1980s, I met Dr. William Gonyea, a professor of anatomy at the University of Texas Southwestern Medical Center. Dr. Gonyea had lifted weights for more than 30 years, and many of his medical students shared his interest in exercise and muscle enlargement.

I was particularly interested in a 6-year study Dr. Gonyea completed with cats. The study was reported in the *Journal of Applied Sport Science Research* (3:85–92, 1989), and the results were intriguing.

Sixty-two cats were conditioned, with a food reward, to lift weights with their right forelimb by performing an exercise resembling a wrist curl.

The cats trained once a day, 5 days per week. All the cats started out lifting 100 grams. The weight was gradually increased as the cats progressed. When a cat failed to make progress after a predetermined period, the muscles of the right and left forelimbs were removed and weighed.

The cats were not forced to perform by punishment.

Thus, the intensity and speed of training was dependent upon each cat's personality and motivation for food. This resulted in a broad range of performance values and muscle-mass increases, which was accounted for with appropriate statistical analyses. Here's how it turned out.

• The cats that eventually trained with the heaviest weights developed larger muscle masses in their exercised forelimbs compared with those that employed lighter weights.

• The cats that used slower lifting speeds developed larger muscles than those using faster lifting speeds.

• Overall, the slower and heavier the lifting, the greater the muscle-mass increase.

Dr. Gonyea is convinced bodybuilders can learn something from his study with cats. Lifting heavy weights slowly is the best way to increase the muscular size of a cat and, he believes, to increase the muscular size of a human.

Weeks 3 and 4: Hitting Smaller Muscles

For weeks 3 and 4, you are going to concentrate on a few smaller, often-neglected muscles. The SuperSlow style will be equally effective with these ignored body parts. Here's the routine.

Smaller-Muscles Routine

1. Hip-adduction machine (If this machine isn't available, use a wide foot spacing on the leg-press machine.)

2. Seated-calf-raise machine

3. Prone back raise on bench

4. Four-way neck machine (If this machine is not available, lie on a bench and have a buddy supply manual resistance to your head in the back and front positions, as described on page 226.)

5. Incline bench press with barbell

6. Bent-over row with barbell

7. Wrist curl with barbell/Reverse wrist curl with barbell

Once again, your Wednesday workout should be NTF. Progress as much as you can, always in good form.

Weeks 5 and 6: Using Negative Only

Negative work is usually more productive than positive work, because you can lower about 40 percent more weight than you can lift. It allows you to make a greater inroad into a muscle's strength and more thoroughly fatigue that muscle. It's also more dangerous. If you do it with loose form, you can overstress your connective tissues and cause injury.

That's why it's important that you perform the following routine with an assistant spotting you on all the recommended exercises. Here are the steps to utilize.

• Increase the weight approximately 40 percent on each negative exercise.

• Get your spotter to help you lift the resistance carefully to the top position. Use machines, if possible, because they're easier and safer to use on negative repetitions.

• Transfer the resistance carefully in the top position and lower it slowly to the bottom. Have your assistant count out 10 seconds as the weight descends.

• Lift the weight quickly, with the spotter's help, back to the top. At first, both the lifting and lowering will be easy. But at repetition 3 or 4, both will become more difficult. Don't stop the set there, however. Focus on relaxing your face and neck.

• Try to complete at least 7 or 8 strict, 8- to 10-second repetitions, with minimum rest between them. If you can do 10 repetitions, you need more resistance.

• Reduce your training from three times a week to twice a week, or four times in 2 weeks.

Negative-Only Routine

1. Leg-extension machine/Leg-curl machine

2. Leg-press machine

3. Lateral-raise machine

4. Overhead-press machine

5. Pullover machine

If you doubt that five exercises will provide enough stimulation for overall growth, you will change your mind after your initial negative-only workout. You'll probably register extreme soreness throughout your body. It should, however, ease a bit after your second workout. By your third workout, your strength will seem to zoom to new levels.

Don't be afraid to tackle some heavy weights; just remember to always be conscious of correct form.

A Week's Layoff

After 6 weeks of progressive training, you'll be wise to take a week off. Another of the basic principles of the do-the-opposite philosophy is that you'll have a rested recovery ability, instead of an exhausted recovery ability. Time away from exercising will help you better prepare for phase IV.

During your week off, keep your daily calorie level the same as during weeks 5 and 6, which should be in the neighborhood of 3,000 per day. Keep drinking a gallon of water and having maintenance doses of creatine monohydrate. The only difference is that you're not training. Rest, relax, and generally take it easy for a week to 10 days.

Hudlow's progress was steady. At the completion of phase III, his body weight had climbed from 192 to 206, for a gain of 14 pounds. After the layoff, he was eager to attack phase IV.

Chapter 28

PHASE IV, CUSTOMIZED WORKOUTS: MIXING, MATCHING, AND MAXING

The bent-arm fly with dumbbells, performed properly, makes a significant inroad into the strength of your chest.

NOW IS THE time to customize your workout to emphasize particular body parts or to work on weak areas. David Hudlow didn't have any unusually weak areas, so we decided to emphasize his biceps, triceps, pectorals, gastrocnemius, quadriceps, and hamstrings. We designed five customized routines, each utilizing some type of pre-exhaustion. (I explained the techniques in chapter 15.)

Note: Perform the bracketed exercises throughout this chapter with minimal rest in between.

You're going to need extra rest to recover from these workouts, which is why I recommend at least 72 hours between all workouts in phase IV. So now you'll be looking at your training in terms of 9-day blocks, rather than neat 7-day weeks.

For example, let's say that your first training block is devoted to your arm routine. You'd do that on Monday, Thursday, and Sunday. After your 72-hour rest, you'd start your chest routine on Wednesday and continue it on Saturday and Tuesday.

The entire specialization course for five body parts requires 6½ weeks, or 45 days. I suggest mapping it all out in advance on a calendar.

Your dietary calories ascend as they did in phase III: 100 calories each 2-week period. If the first week of specialized training is labeled "Week 8," then the calories progress as follows:

- 3,100 calories per day for weeks 8 and 9

- 3,200 calories per day for weeks 10 and 11

- 3,300 calories per day for weeks 12 and 13

- 3,400 calories per day for week 14

Your creatine monohydrate maintenance and water drinking remain the same as in phase III.

Arm Routine: Emphasizing Full Development

Here's the triceps and biceps workout that is guaranteed to get your attention.

Triceps: Double Pre-Exhaustion

1. Slow 1½-repetition dip: 30-second negative, 30-second positive, 30-second negative

2. Lying triceps extension with barbell

3. Dip, negative only

Biceps: Double Pre-Exhaustion

4. Slow 1½-repetition chinup: 30-second negative, 30-second positive, 30-second negative

5. Biceps curl with dumbbells

6. Chinup, negative only

7. Standing-calf-raise machine

8. Leg-press machine

You'll need access to parallel bars for dipping and a horizontal bar for chinning. The Nautilus multi-exercise machine is great for both. A friend with a watch that has a second hand is also a must.

You start both 1½-repetition exercises (dip and chinup) in the top position, take a full 30 seconds to lower your body to the stretched position, then a full 30 seconds to move back to the top, and another 30 seconds to the bottom. Those 90-second sets are grueling. Your friend can help by calling out your time as you move through each 30-second segment.

After completing the 1½-repetition exercises, immediately move to the single-joint exercises. These are two new exercises, but you should know how to do them. Keep the style smooth (about a 4-second positive and a 4-second negative), and try to do at least 8 reps. Then, quickly get to the negative-only dip or chinup. A chair, box, or stairs under the parallel bars or chinning bar will allow your legs to do the positive portion of these exercises. Climb into the top position, remove your feet and stabilize your body, and lower slowly to the stretched position. Climb quickly back to the top and repeat the slow lowering. Your objective is at least 8 repetitions.

Push yourself on both of these double pre-exhaustion cycles, and you'll get a terrific pump. Rest for several minutes and proceed to the calf raise and leg press.

That's it—your entire workout should take only 20 minutes or less.

And remember, rest 72 hours before you repeat the arm routine. Hit it three times in 9 days, and then get ready for the chest routine.

Chest Routine: Expanding and Deepening Your Pectorals

These two pre-exhaustion cycles will shock your pectorals to new growth.

Upper Chest: Pre-Exhaustion

1. Incline bent-arm fly with dumbbells

2. Incline bench press with barbell

Middle Chest: Pre-Exhaustion

3. Bent-arm fly with dumbbells

4. Bench press with barbell

5. Biceps curl with barbell

6. Leg-extension machine

7. Leg-curl machine

8. Four-way neck machine

Do the four chest exercises listed above in a smooth, slow style and grind out as many repetitions as possible. Resist bouncing in and out of those stretched positions. Make your pectorals do the work.

Back Routine: Flaring Your Lats

The back routine features a pre-exhaustion cycle followed by a double pre-exhaustion grouping, guaranteed to give your lats an intense workout.

Lats: Pre-Exhaustion

1. Straight-arm pullover with one dumbbell

2. Behind-the-neck pulldown on lat machine

Lats: Double Pre-Exhaustion

3. Bent-over row with barbell

4. Bent-arm pullover with barbell

5. Chinup, negative only

6. Shoulder shrug with barbell

7. Leg-extension machine

8. Squat with barbell

Calf Routine: Stressing the Stretch

Many bodybuilders neglect the stretched position when they perform the calf raise. This is a mistake.

Here's a cycle that not only directs you to emphasize the stretched position on all your calf raises but also asks you to hold the last repetition at the bottom for 30 seconds. You're going to feel these like never before.

Calves: Double Pre-Exhaustion

1. Standing-calf-raise machine, with 30-second stretch on last repetition

2. Leg-curl machine

3. Standing-calf-raise machine, with 30-second stretch on last repetition

4. Lateral raise with dumbbells

5. Straight-arm pullover with one dumbbell

6. Dip, negative only

7. Leg-extension machine/Leg-press machine

The standing calf raise is best accomplished on a machine that supplies a movement arm and a stable step for the balls of your feet. Be sure to keep your knees locked as you elevate your heel slowly to the contracted position. Pause, lower smoothly, and repeat for maximum repetitions. On the final repetition, hold in the stretched position for 30 seconds. To help dissipate the pain, relax your face and focus on your breathing.

Thigh Routine: Concentrating on Thickness

For thick, muscular thighs, you must perform full-range movements and adhere to correct form in all the recommended exercises. This workout involves a quadriceps cycle and a hamstrings cycle. It also applies a 30-second stretch on the last repetition of each thigh exercise.

Quadriceps: Pre-Exhaustion

1. Leg-extension machine, with 30-second stretch on last repetition

2. Leg-press machine, with 30-second stretch on last repetition

Hamstrings: Pre-Exhaustion

3. Leg-curl machine, with 30-second stretch on last repetition

4. Stiff-legged deadlift with barbell, with 30-second stretch on last repetition

5. Seated-calf-raise machine

6. Bent-over row with barbell/Pulldown on lat machine

7. Bench press with barbell

You'll need a buddy to help count you through those 30-second stretches on the four thigh exercises. Try not to allow the resistance to touch the weight stack on the machine movements. A half-inch distance will work well. Even if the weight touches, keep the tension on the targeted muscle.

Do your best to relax your face and regulate your breathing. Doing so will allow you to get maximum growth from this intense training. Work hard, and you'll be surprised by your results.

Hudlow's Results

In any long-term bodybuilding project, sooner or later you must deal with such things as home responsibilities, work and educational conflicts, financial problems, interpersonal relationships, and sicknesses. In other words, the stresses of everyday living can add up and have a detrimental effect on your bodybuilding.

David Hudlow's Physical Transformation

In approximately 4 months, David Hudlow added 2³⁄₈ inches onto each biceps, 6 inches onto his chest, and 3³⁄₈ inches onto each thigh.

Results of Phase I

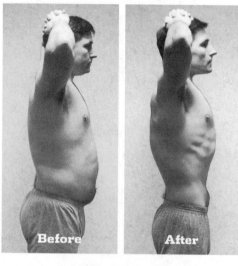

Lost 50 pounds of fat.

Results of Phase II

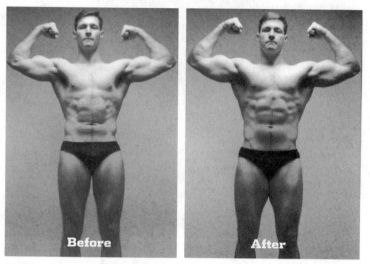

Built 18½ pounds of muscle.

Results of Phases III and IV

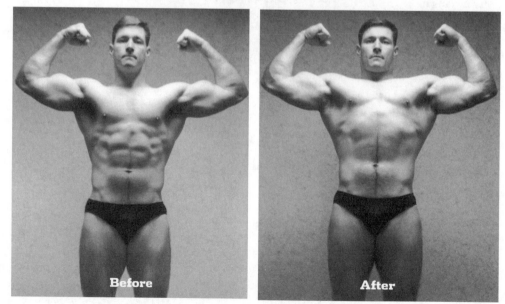

Gained 23 pounds of mass.

During the third week of phase IV, David Hudlow came down with what we thought was a head cold. He missed a workout. By the next scheduled workout, however, the cold turned out to be the flu. He missed another two training sessions. Then, he started final examinations in his classes at the University of Florida, which meant he would be lacking in sleep for at least a week.

Hudlow, an ex-marine, didn't want to admit that the illnesses and lack of sleep were affecting his progress. But they were. Prior to his illness, his body weight had increased from 206 to 208, then to 211, and finally to a high of 216 pounds. After the sickness and final exams, he was back to 206. He had probably lost most of the new muscle he built during the arm and chest routines.

We had two choices: Either take a break and then begin again with the first specialized workout or pick up where we left off. We decided on the latter.

During the last two body parts, calves and thighs, Hudlow made good progress. He completed phase IV weighing 215, for a gain of 9 pounds. I'm confident that he would have weighed 220 pounds or more if he hadn't gotten sick.

Nevertheless, during phases III and IV, Hudlow gained 23 pounds, although our calculations showed that $6\frac{1}{2}$ of those pounds were fat. So he actually built $16\frac{1}{2}$ pounds of muscle during phases III and IV. He also increased each arm by 1 inch, his chest by $3\frac{3}{8}$ inches, each thigh by $1\frac{3}{4}$ inches, and each calf by $\frac{1}{2}$ inch.

If you compare the photo of Hudlow at the conclusion of phase II with the one taken after phase IV, the size gain is unmistakable. But he's clearly not as lean after phase IV as he'd been at the end of phase II. That's why he spent the month following

phase IV on fat loss. His strategy was pretty simple: cut calories.

The Final Numbers

Here's what Hudlow accomplished in 6 months (all fractions have been rounded to the nearest whole number).

- Began at a body weight of 219 pounds

- Lost 50 pounds of fat and built 5 pounds of muscle (phase I, 66 days)

- Built 18 pounds of muscle (phase II, 14 days)

- Built 16 pounds of muscle and regained 6 pounds of fat (phase III and IV, 87 days)

- Transformed his body composition dramatically by losing 44 pounds of fat and building 39 pounds of muscle

- Ended the course weighing 215 pounds but looking much different than 6 months earlier

Do-the-Opposite Philosophy

You can succeed in transforming your body with this philosophy. In the process, you can help turn bodybuilding right side up. Here are the most important concepts.

- Intensity, not duration
- Briefer, not longer, workouts
- Infrequent, not daily, training
- Rest, not more sets
- Slow, not fast repetitions
- Smooth, not jerky, movements
- Superhydration, not dehydration
- Carbohydrate-rich, not protein-rich, diet
- Creatine, not drugs

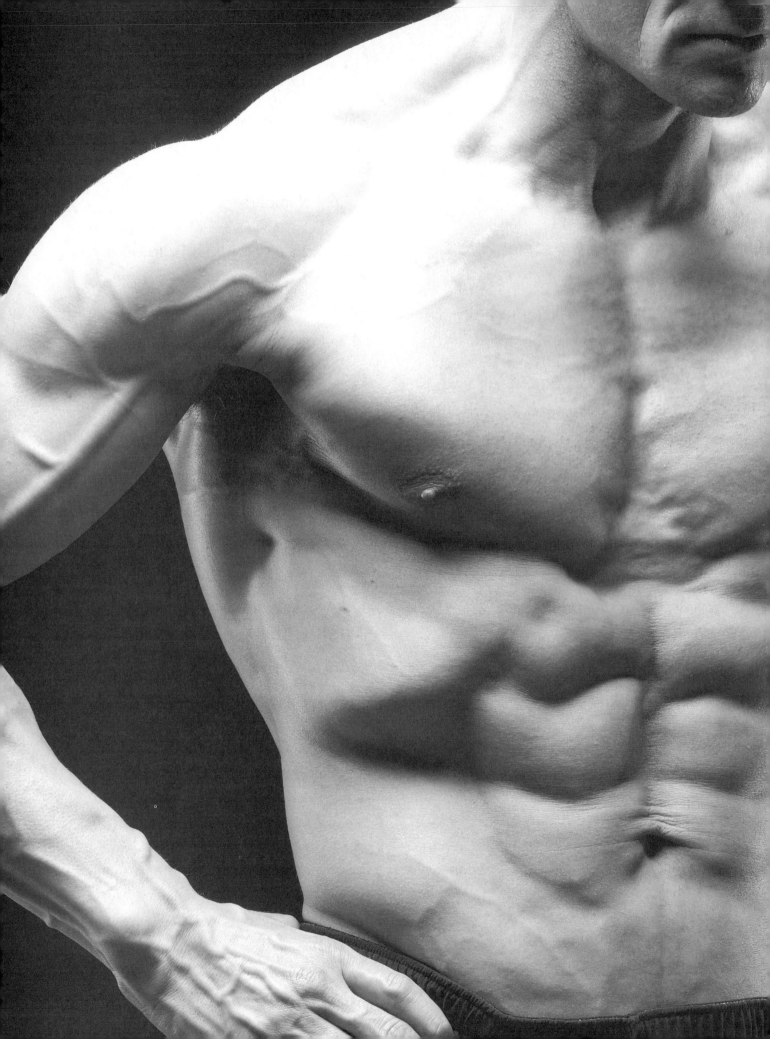

PART VI

HIT QUESTIONS, ANSWERS, AND TRENDS

Attention to detail, hard work, and persistence are important prerequisites in building your body effectively and efficiently with the new HIT.

Chapter 29

THE HIT SQUAD:
ADDRESSING CRITICISM

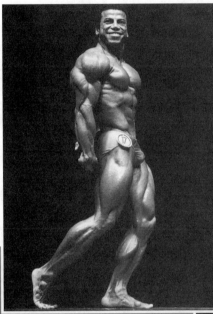

Chris Dickerson, 1970
Mr. America and 1982
Mr. Olympia, had the
best calves I've ever
seen on a bodybuilder—
and their size and shape
were primarily because
of his long soleus and
gastrocnemius muscles.
Dickerson had an
identical twin brother,
who was not into
bodybuilding, and his
calves were also
unusually large and
impressive from zero
training.

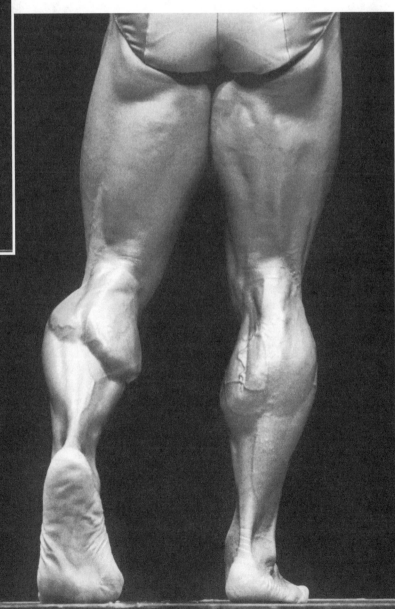

FROM TIME TO time, HIT takes a few hits. Here are some of the major criticisms, along with my rebuttals.

HIT: For Beginners Only?

Question: I keep hearing that HIT is okay for beginners but not for advanced bodybuilding. Advanced bodybuilders must do a lot of different exercises for shaping and plenty of sets for pumping. What's your opinion?

Answer: Yeah, I've heard the same things. If a beginner, for example, continued with HIT and never decreased his duration and frequency, then such a plateau is likely to happen. So for HIT to be effective for 6 months to a year, you must chip away at both the duration and frequency, as well as some of the intensity with an occasional not-to-failure (NTF) workout. All of this is explained in part III.

As for doing more exercises and more sets to facilitate shaping and pumping, I disagree. Muscular shape is not determined by so-called angle training, as much as it is by genetics. And though muscular pumping certainly feels powerful to some degree, it is not a requirement for growth stimulation.

HIT, properly planned and properly performed, works effectively for beginner, intermediate, and advanced bodybuilders.

Returning to High-Volume Training (HVT)

Question: According to a certain muscle magazine, some champion bodybuilders have used HIT, but they almost always return to HVT. Why?

Answer: It's difficult to speak for these cham-

pions, and who knows if such interviews actually took place or not. As I've stated previously, champion bodybuilders are rare breeds. Often, how they train has little to do with how they look.

No one, however, argues with the fact that HIT, properly performed, is hard work. It requires the utmost focus, determination, and motivation for best results. In truth, the average bodybuilder has more to gain from HIT than does the champion. The champion, with favorable genetics in his corner, can stumble, do haphazard repetitions, and overtrain, but still look decent. The typical bodybuilder, however, needs to have everything going in his favor to click on the muscular-growth process successfully.

Not everyone has the necessary attitude, drive, and patience to sustain HIT continuously for a year or two. That's why it's important to take frequent layoffs, utilize NTF workouts, and decrease your overall duration and frequency of exercising.

My question to many champion bodybuilders is this: If it actually does require 2 to 3 hours a day of training, 5 or 6 days a week (10 to 18 hours a week devoted to training), for a minimum of 5 years or longer to build a championship physique, is it actually worth it?

I think not.

Is One Set to Failure for Everybody?

Question: Are you saying that one-set-to-failure HIT works for everybody? If so, why are there so many bodybuilders into HVT?

Answer: One set to failure works only for those people who truly know how to go to failure in good form. A lot of bodybuilders don't. As I've explained multiple times throughout this book, failure is not an easy concept to achieve consistently in good form.

Think of the bell-shaped curve that applies to a random selection of 100 trainees, which normally subdivide into three groups. On the left is a small group of 16 bodybuilders. On the right is another small group of 16. In the middle, under the primary curve, is a large group of 68 bodybuilders.

Here's the way I see going to failure, today. Out of every group of 100 bodybuilders, you'll find 16 of them that can go to failure on their own accord. But there will also be an equal-sized group of 16 who, for whatever reason or reasons, cannot go to failure. Then you have the 68 bodybuilders in the middle who, with the right instruction and motivation, can probably learn to go to failure.

The small group on the left includes the guys who contribute to the HIT Web sites and chat rooms you find on the Internet. The small group on the right engage in the high-volume training (HVT) Internet sites. And often, the groups tie into one another in no-holds-barred verbal battles. It's sometimes fascinating to read the back-and-forth arguments.

All that bickering is probably healthy, if not too time-consuming. But the primary group that this book is intended for is the large one in the middle, the 68 percent of the bodybuilders who are unsure about HIT, who aren't familiar with it, or who most certainly need help organizing, planning, and applying it to their weekly strength training.

In reality, as I was explaining in the introduction of this book, that 16 percent on the left who were at one time enthusiastically into HIT has significantly shrunk, let's say by 50 percent. On the other hand, the HVT group has increased by 50 percent. So, using our same numbers, out of our selected 100 bodybuilders, the HIT group on the left has decreased to 8, the HVT on the right has grown to 24, and the large group in the middle remains unchanged at 68.

From what I observe in my research and travels, HIT is not as popular today as it was in 1990. And HVT is more popular today than it was in 1990. One of my primary objectives in writing this book is to supply the old and new HIT people with noteworthy facts, routines, and stories to renew their enthusiasm and improve their results. In the process, just maybe some of that large group of bodybuilders in the middle will be willing to give some of the HIT routines in this book a fair trial.

Back to the question: Does one set to failure work for everyone? Of course not; some trainees simply don't have the mindset to go to all-out failure consistently. Remember chapter 5, when Arthur Jones tried to push Arnold Schwarzenegger? For whatever reason(s), Arnold didn't want to train with such intensity. So one set to failure won't work for all trainees, but it will work for most.

Why are so many bodybuilders involved with HVT? HVT is easier to do and certainly easier to understand. HVT is primarily pushed by the leading bodybuilding magazines, so it gets much more publicity than HIT. And the more-is-better philosophy makes better sense in our society, which as a whole is surrounded by all kinds of more-is-better thinking.

Even under ideal circumstances, I doubt that HIT will ever be as popular as HVT.

Duplicating the Results of Viator and Hudlow

Question: I'm fascinated by reading about Casey Viator and David Hudlow putting on all that muscle so quickly. Are you saying that with the HIT routines in this book, I could do the same thing with my body?

Answer: What I'm saying is that the HIT routines, properly practiced, will move you closer to reaching your genetic potential in the muscle-building department than will HVT routines. But after 6 months of HIT, will your body look like

Viator's or Hudlow's? That depends almost entirely on your genetics.

Here's something we used to talk about at the Nautilus plant in Lake Helen. After Viator won the Mr. America in 1971, some of his family visited Lake Helen. His parents were large-boned people, but the Viator everyone talked about was his older sister. She was about Casey's height and weighed a solid 180 pounds. And she'd never trained at all.

Sergio Oliva said that he had a brother in Cuba who was almost as big and strong but who'd never done any weight training. All he did was cut sugarcane.

Chris Dickerson, Mr. America 1970, had perhaps the best calves ever. Yet he had a twin brother who

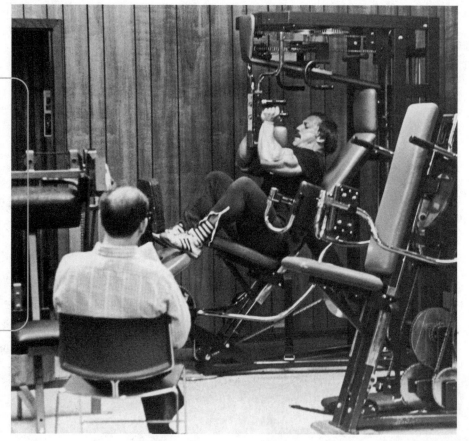

From a competitive-bodybuilding career that stretched 27 years, Casey Viator has tried just about every system of training. But he will tell you honestly that his absolute best gains were made when he was under the HIT tutelage of Arthur Jones in the early 1970s.

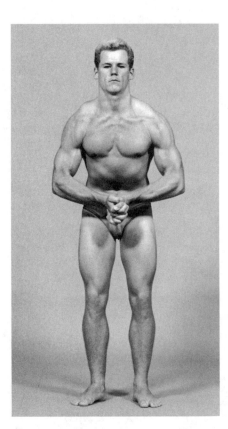 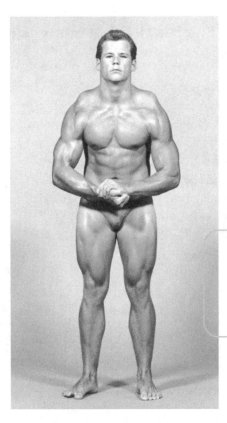

Eddie Mueller had the potential to add 18 pounds of muscle to his body, and he did so in a 10-week HIT plan.

wasn't into bodybuilding but whose calves were just as impressive.

My point is that you must have the inherited capabilities to build muscle quickly. Some people have them; most people don't. But all of us can increase, improve, and perfect what we have.

Another interesting point: The bodybuilders I've trained who built the most muscle in 6 weeks—Jeff Turner (18 pounds), David Hammond (22 pounds), Keith Whitley (29 pounds), and David Hudlow (34 pounds)—weren't completely satisfied. Each still wanted more muscle. Perhaps you or I would have been satisfied with 20 to 30 pounds of added muscle, but not them. In fact, none of the champions I've talked with—Viator, Oliva, Boyer Coe, Mike Mentzer—was ever satis-

fied with his own physique. More muscle was never enough.

But more muscle is a start. The HIT routines in this book will help you get as big as you can, as quickly as you can—within the framework of your genetic potential.

Potential for Adding Muscle

Question: How do you determine your potential for adding a lot of muscle to your body?

Answer: Generally, you must have muscle to build muscle. You can't build it on your forehead or ankles, because you don't have muscle there. That was my point in chapter 7, when I showed you how to measure the length of your biceps and triceps muscles to judge their growth potential.

The Most Dangerous Repetition

Most bodybuilders believe they can avoid injury if they terminate a set prior to the most difficult repetitions, which they consider the most dangerous. In fact, the opposite is true. The further you progress into a set, the safer the work becomes.

Regardless of the number of repetitions involved in a set, the first repetition is the most dangerous, and the last repetition is the safest. The more difficult it feels, the safer it is. The more dangerous it seems, the safer it is.

Here's why: When you lift, you don't feel your actual output. Instead, you feel the percentage of your possible output at that moment. If you can press 200 pounds, then 100 will feel light to you during the first repetition but heavier during each following repetition. By the time you reach a point at which could do just one more repetition, the 100 pounds will feel very heavy. And it should: At that point, you need 100 percent of your strength to move it.

The chance of injury isn't related directly to those feelings of relative strength or exhaustion within a set. Your connective tissues—where injuries are most likely to occur—react according to the actual weight being lifted and the acceleration of that weight. Let's say that a par-

ticular tendon can withstand 100 units of pull but might tear if you forced it to pull against 105 units. Its ability to withstand 100 units doesn't change throughout a set. Whether it's the first repetition or the 12th, that tendon can still withstand 100 units.

But muscles are different. The muscles pulling on the tendon might be able to exert 200 units of pull. If they did so, they would surely injure the tendon. But with each repetition in a set, the muscles' ability to exert force decreases. So if you do 12 repetitions in which the muscles exert 100 units of pull, the muscles exhaust themselves to the point at which 100 units is truly their maximum. But the set never forces the connective tissues to deal with forces they can't handle.

Unfortunately, most bodybuilders avoid the most-productive repetitions in all their sets because of an unjustified fear of injury. After working right up to the point at which only 1 more repetition is possible, they stop, thus avoiding the safest repetition of all, and the only one capable of producing the maximum growth stimulation they seek.

Longer muscles have more potential than do shorter muscles.

Here are a few more signs that you have the genetic underpinnings for a big muscle gain.

• A natural thickness in your major muscle groups, especially your upper arms, forearms, and calves

• A draping shape in your latissimus dorsi muscles and thickness in your upper pectorals

• Unusual roundness in the vastus medialis muscle above your knee (the one that's shaped like a teardrop) and roundness throughout your hamstrings

• Thickness in your lower back and gluteals

Once you've been looking at muscles long enough, you can spot genetic potential for muscle growth almost immediately. You can even see the signs on guys who've never lifted a weight.

Lack of Potential

Question: What if I look in the mirror and don't see any roundness or thickness in the muscles you mentioned? Should I stop trying?

Answer: It's great that you want to put on some muscular size and strength, but I think it's healthy to be realistic in your assessments and goals. Bodybuilding magazines lead you to believe that anyone can look like Flex Wheeler, Ronnie Coleman, Jay Cutler, or whoever is the current champion. Of course, according to the magazines, not only do you need to train the way the champions do, which is HVT, but you need to subscribe to their dietary-supplement schedule.

A little history: In the 1960s, the major bodybuilding magazines—Bob Hoffman's *Strength and Health* and Joe Weider's *Muscle Builder/Power*—realized there was little money in selling barbells and dumbbells. You didn't get many repeat sales from a barbell set, and the shipping costs were fairly high. But supplements and health foods presented a more interesting opportunity. They could be made and shipped cheaply, and by their nature they led to repeat orders. And the magazines were perfect vehicles for promoting them. It cost nothing to mention them in articles and relatively little to get bodybuilding champions to endorse them. So protein powders and pills turned into a very lucrative endeavor.

Since the early 1900s, the muscle magazines were pushers of hope—hope for bigger, stronger muscles; hope for more vim and vigor. Now with the protein supplements, they had something else to reinforce that hope. They stopped telling readers that exercise was responsible for 80 percent of their results. Instead, they said that results were 80 percent dependent on nutrition, especially from protein.

Hoffman and Weider started something in the 1960s that still has not abated. In fact, the profits today in nutritional supplements related to bodybuilding are astronomically high.

One thing I always admired about Arthur Jones was that he never bought into nutritional supplements. If he had, it would have surely meant instant profits for Nautilus Sports/Medical Industries. He thought the entire nutritional-supplement industry was based on selling false hope. Jones was completely honest with every bodybuilder who visited him. He always gave each man his sincere opinion of his physique and bodybuilding potential. Then he supplied realistic hope, as opposed to false hope.

Many were temporarily upset, especially if they'd been bodybuilding for 5 years or longer and Jones told them that their hoped-for physique was simply impossible. But months or years later, many of them would return and thank him for helping them reassess their lives for the better.

One of my goals in writing this book is to provide the necessary tools for a realistic evaluation of your bodybuilding potential.

Build as much muscle as you can in a healthy manner. Extra muscle will help you in many ways. But becoming a successful bodybuilder, to the point of entering competition, that's another thing altogether. You must have long muscles throughout your body to compete successfully, and that's 100 percent inherited.

Without those inherited traits, you can still build your body. But forget about winning a major bodybuilding show. It's simply not going to happen. That doesn't mean you can't get a pretty darn good physique—because you can. And it won't take you all that long if you apply the concepts in this book.

So work hard and be realistic.

Anabolic Steroids

Question: It sure looks to me like both Viator and Hudlow were on anabolic steroids. Were they?

Answer: Jones would have killed Viator if

there was even a hint of him being on steroids. So, no, Viator was not on steroids when he trained with Jones. And neither was Hudlow when I worked with him in Gainesville.

As I mentioned in the introduction of this book, anabolic steroids, growth hormone, and other drugs have just about ruined the competitive sport of bodybuilding in the United States. If these drugs had existed to the same degree in the 1950s, 1960s, and 1970s as they do today, the competitors would probably have been similarly involved. Let's face it, competitive athletes, especially bodybuilders, are easy marks for purveyors of hope—and drugs certainly provide hope. Unfortunately, few people realize that thousands of guys take drugs and still don't look good. Yes, certain drugs, stacked together in large amounts, help some men build muscle and recover faster—while subjecting their bodies to potentially damaging side effects. Furthermore, most of this drug taking by bodybuilders is self-administered and not supervised by medical doctors, so the situation is even more dangerous. Today, the simple unlawful possession of anabolic steroids is a third-degree felony in all 50 states. Of course, you must be caught and convicted.

The best advice I have concerning bodybuilding drugs is: Don't get involved. And if you are involved, seek qualified help immediately.

Chapter 30

HIT BITS:
SMOOTHING ROUGH EDGES

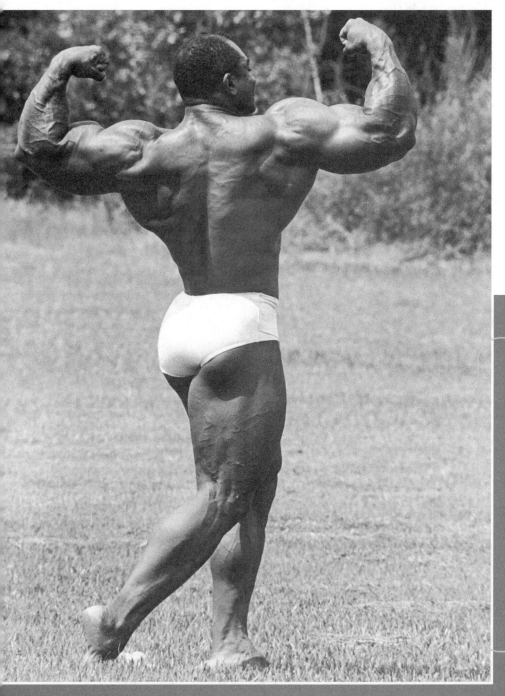

The accurate measuring of Sergio Oliva's arms, before and after his workouts, taught Arthur Jones that the closer you get to reaching your genetic potential for size in your biceps and triceps, the less muscular pump you achieve from any amount of exercise. Because Oliva's arms were as big as they could get, their circumference did *not* increase after a hard workout.

IN THIS BOOK I've covered a lot of topics, some only briefly. This often opens the door for misunderstandings. This chapter addresses some of those concerns.

HIT Split Routines

Question: What's the best way to split the normal HIT routine into upper body one day and lower body the next?

Answer: The best way is not to split the routine. I've experimented with various splits: upper body/lower body, pushing/pulling, legs/torso/arms, abdominals/legs/torso/arms, and even one called contra-lateral, which involved the left upper body and right lower body on one day and the right upper body and left lower body on another day. Generally, after 3 or 4 weeks, all these split routines led to overtraining. Why? Because split routines, compared with the whole-body routines in this book, always involve more total exercises per 2-week period.

Indirect Effect

Question: Without split routines, my fear is that I just won't be able to work all my major muscles thoroughly. Any advice?

Answer: You don't have to work all your major muscles thoroughly at each workout. Over a 2-week period, yes. But doing so each workout would lead to overtraining.

Plus there's a concept known as the indirect effect. A hard set of chinups, for example, will not only work your biceps and lats, but you'll also feel it in the surrounding muscles—your forearms, neck, pectorals, trapezius, and abdominals. The squat with a barbell hits your quadriceps, buttocks, and hamstrings directly but also has an indirect effect on your lower back and calves, and even your upper body.

Put another way, the more you focus on multiple-joint exercises, such as the chinup and squat, the less you have to worry about single-joint exercises that target individual muscles.

Multiple-Joint or Single-Joint Exercises

Question: Are multiple-joint exercises more important than single-joint exercises?

Answer: If you had to make a choice between the two, then yes, multiple-joint exercises are more important than single-joint movements. But doing both is almost always better than doing either one exclusively. How would you effectively work the vastus medialis of your front thigh without a leg-extension machine? You can't. The same thing is true when you're trying to address the muscles of your neck and calves. There is definitely a place for single-joint exercises in bodybuilding.

Neck Exercises

Question: How do I work my neck if I don't have access to a four-way neck machine?

Answer: Your best bet here is to team up with a partner/spotter and let him provide hand/arm resistance against your moving head. The most important positions are neck extension and neck flexion. Here's a description of how to perform each.

Back Neck Extension

• Lie facedown on a low bench or table with your chin and head off the end of the bench.

• Have the spotter kneel to your right side and place his right hand securely on the back of your head and his left hand in the middle of your back. The right hand supplies resistance to your moving head, and the left hand adds stability to your torso.

• Extend your head upward and backward as the spotter applies only a little resistance at first, until you get the hang of what to expect.

• Lower your head slowly until your chin is near your chest. Again the spotter supplies resistance to the back of your head so that you get benefits from the negative part of the repetition.

• Continue doing the movements. After 3 or 4 repetitions, it's the spotter's job to increase the resistance to stimulate an all-out effort. But be extra careful initially, because your neck is a vulnerable area.

• Perform from 8 to 12 repetitions and move to the front flexion.

Front Neck Flexion

• Lie on your back on a low bench or table with your head off the end of the bench.

• Have your spotter kneel to your left side and place the palm of his left hand under your chin and his right hand low on your forehead. Both his left and right hands supply resistance to your flexing head.

• Begin with your head extended backward so that your neck is fully stretched.

• Move your head upward and forward as the spotter provides a little resistance to your chin. Try to move only your head and not your shoulders.

• Continue doing the repetitions smoothly and slowly. After 4 repetitions, the spotter makes the movement harder in both the positive and negative phases.

• Do 8 to 12 repetitions.

Think safety first when exercising your neck. Don't get into a competition with your spotter during this movement. Keep each repetition slow and smooth and avoid any jerky movement.

Muscular Pumping

Question: I've applied HIT for many years with good results, but one thing has always puzzled me. I don't seem to get as much of a muscular pump as I used to. Can you tell me why?

Answer: Yes, I noticed the same thing. Evidently, as you move closer and closer to reaching your full potential, a muscular pump serves little purpose. In fact, I remember Arthur Jones demonstrating this to me during one of Sergio Oliva's workouts in 1971. Before the workout, Jones measured Oliva's contracted right upper arm at 20⅛ inches.

Jones had Oliva do leg and torso cycles before he worked his arms. His arm routine consisted of the biceps curl with a barbell, Nautilus biceps curl, Nautilus triceps extension, and wrist curl with a barbell. Afterward, Jones had Oliva lie on his back on the floor with his arms outstretched, to make it easier for the blood to reach his arms. After 90 seconds, he had him stand up and contract his right arm again for a measurement.

Sweat was everywhere, Oliva's veins were in bold relief, and his biceps and triceps were pumped to massive proportions. He could just barely flex his elbow, and his right arm appeared several inches larger.

Muscles: The Rat Race

Exercise scientists will tell you that muscle growth depends on the availability of certain hormones, and that no growth will occur if there isn't adequate nutrition. But an intriguing 1975 study performed on laboratory rats showed otherwise. The work was done by Dr. Alfred L. Goldberg and colleagues and was reported in *Medicine and Science in Sports* (7: 248–261, 1975).

Dr. Goldberg and his researchers surgically cut the gastrocnemius muscles of one leg in one group of rats. Since the gastrocnemius is the most important muscle for working the ankle joint in walking and running (as well as in strength exercises like the standing calf raise), the rats now had to compensate for the missing muscle by using two other ankle muscles, the plantaris and soleus.

As expected, when the rats ran on a treadmill, the plantaris and soleus muscles on their surgically altered legs grew dramatically, compared with the same muscles on their unaltered legs.

In the next phase of the research, surgically altered rats were given other handicaps. One group had a procedure to prevent them from producing growth hormone. Another group couldn't produce insulin. Another was put on a starvation diet in which they received only water.

Other groups had various combinations of those procedures.

Then all the animals ran on treadmills. When the exercise portion was finished and the rats were examined, it showed that all the surgically altered rats had bigger plantaris and soleus muscles. Those muscles grew on a starvation diet, without insulin, and without growth hormone. They grew at the expense of other body tissues, and in spite of the fact that their growth and consumption of resources meant a loss of health.

Here's the key: Even though the rats' total weight and muscle mass fell some 30 percent, the plantaris and soleus muscles actually increased in size and weight. The researchers had stumbled onto a fundamental biological priority: If stimulated, muscle will grow in spite of tremendous adversity and at the expense of the remainder of the organism.

What does that mean for you? Probably this: The rat muscles grew because they were needed for locomotion; without locomotion, the rats would've died. So if you want your muscles to grow, you must convince your body that growth is vital. Your muscles must be stimulated and forced to grow through hard, brief, and infrequent exercise.

Arthur called me to step forward for a closer look. The paper-thin tape was around his arm and it read 20⅛ inches—exactly the same as before.

Jones went on to explain that he had measured Oliva's arm several times previously under similar conditions, with identical results. Yes, Oliva felt pumped, and he looked pumped. But the measurement wasn't larger.

Once you reach your full potential in a particular muscle, such as the biceps and triceps, Jones reasoned, there's no place for the excessive blood and fluids to go—at least, not in that particular muscle. Maybe the blood pools near the joints,

where it's difficult to measure, as opposed to the muscle bellies. That would explain why an arm that feels and looks pumped is no bigger than it was cold.

Jones concluded that the size of your arm when fully pumped represents its growth potential. So if your arms are an inch larger when fully pumped, they have the potential to grow at least an inch.

High-Protein Eating and Bodybuilding

Question: You mentioned earlier that a high-protein diet isn't necessary to build muscle. So how come just about everyone connected with body-building believes the opposite?

Answer: From 1970 to 1973, I studied nutrition at Florida State University with Dr. Harold Schendel, who had spent a number of years in Africa working with starving children. I remember him telling me about how his team of doctors initially rushed into a famine country, assembled the starving children, and tried to force-feed them high-protein diets. Rather than improve, their conditions got worse. They quickly realized that what these children needed were calories. The more simple the carbohydrates were that they gave them, the more they improved. What worked best was a mush mixture of water, sugar, and fatty acids, with very small amounts of protein, vitamins, and minerals.

Later in his career, Dr. Schendel studied amino acids and had a hand in establishing the Recommended Dietary Allowances for protein. In 1970, he convinced me to do a 2-month study on my body to determine if massive protein intake was beneficial. I was consuming more than 300 grams of protein a day back then. I kept accurate records of my food intake and activity for 60 days, and I even collected all my urine for the same period. Afterward, I used the Kjeldahl method for determining nitrogen in my urine, which is a measure of protein utilization.

To my surprise, any time I consumed more than the RDA of protein, the excess was excreted in my urine. Dr. Schendel concluded that my kidneys were working overtime to metabolize the excess protein. He also explained that human kidneys and livers show overuse symptoms in the presence of massive amounts of protein. We know from long-term animal studies that high-protein diets will shorten life spans.

So I stopped my massive protein diet and immediately felt a surge of energy from unburdening my kidneys and liver.

In the 1970s, the daily recommendation for protein was 0.36 gram of protein per pound of body weight. In other words, if you weigh 200 pounds, you would need 72 grams of protein a day—a couple of chicken breasts. Yet, when I weighed 200 pounds, I was eating 300 grams of protein a day, more than four times the recommended amount. About half of those 300 grams came from my four daily protein shakes.

Of course, I'd been greatly influenced by reading the muscle magazines and their cleverly designed collections of editorials, articles, and advertisements that promoted protein supplements and high-protein eating.

I recommend no more than 0.36 gram of protein per pound of body weight a day. For most lifters, that means about 10 to 20 percent of your total calories will come from protein. I also recommend that about 20 to 30 percent of your calories come from fat, and about 60 to 70 percent from carbohydrates. I've used this formula with every bodybuilder I've trained.

The facts show that you simply do not require much protein to build muscle. Human muscle is at least 70 percent water. Only 20 percent of muscle is protein. Because muscle is mostly water, 1 pound of muscle contains only 600 calories. Calories and water are more important to the muscle-building process than is protein.

But if you are the publisher of a leading bodybuilding magazine, from a promotional, money-making point of view, how much revenue could you produce from pushing calories and water? Calories and water are everywhere, at least in the United States. But as a sales pitch, "calories and water" doesn't have the magic of these:

• "Premium micro, ultra filtration, whey protein"

• "Advanced protein synthesis complex"

• "100% enzymatically digested bioactive protein isolate"

While Oliva was training in Florida in 1971, his favorite meal was pepperoni pizza, washed down with 32 ounces of Coca-Cola—not exactly what I'd call a high-protein meal. But it was more than adequate in calories and water.

How Much Protein Is Enough?

Question: It's not just the muscle magazines that suggest eating more protein. Most sports nutritionists today recommend from 0.6 to 0.8 gram of protein per pound of body weight. Did you disagree with them, too?

Answer: There's been some research over the past 10 years showing that *perhaps* there are advantages for power athletes and bodybuilders to consume 50 to 100 percent more protein than the RDA of 0.36 gram of protein per pound of body weight. I don't buy into it—not completely, anyway.

Here's what I do believe: Only intense exercise generates cellular messages that stimulate DNA to begin the process of expanding muscle fibers. An excess of dietary protein, or other nutrients, won't generate these messages. Nutrition enters the picture only after the muscles are stimulated to grow. And even then, rest is at least as equally important as nutrition.

I'm not against a little extra protein in your diet.

Just don't go completely overboard and bump it up to three or four times the RDA. Consuming 250 to 300 grams of protein per day—whether it's from food or supplements—is expensive, wasteful, and not the safest thing you could do for your liver and kidneys.

Is 1,500 Calories per Day Too Low?

Question: I've been doing HIT on and off since college. Today, I'm 32, 6 feet 3 inches, and 260 pounds. I know I've got some fat to lose, but the 1,500 calories a day in your quick-start plan seems skimpy. Can I add a few calories to the plan?

Answer: Yes. If you're taller than 6 feet 2 and weigh 250 or more, you need about 300 more calories per day. One simple way to do this is to add four slices of whole wheat bread to the recommended 1,500-calories-per-day menus. Whole wheat bread is an excellent food, with 70 percent carbohydrate, 17 percent protein, and 13 percent fat. Or if you'd rather have a 300-calorie meal-replacement shake, that's fine, too. Just make sure you read the label and make appropriate adjustments to get to 300 calories.

Some extremely active men who weigh less than 250 pounds will also require those 300 extra calories a day. These include men who work outside in demanding jobs, such as construction, loading and unloading, or plumbing. Guys who work two jobs a day may also fall into this category.

You'll probably know that you require more calories per day during the second week of the plan. You'll feel very fatigued, and the strength training will seem too difficult. If this happens to you, increase your calories by 300 per day.

Sweating and Fat Loss

Question: Will working up a good sweat during HIT help me lose more fat?

Answer: Sweating won't help you lose body fat, though it may temporarily reduce your weight. Weight loss from sweat is depletion of water, not fat. As soon as you quench your thirst, your weight usually returns to normal.

Excessive sweating can cause your body to start preserving fat. You should particularly avoid rubber sweat suits, belts, and wraps. Even steam, sauna, and whirlpool baths can lead to problems.

Ideally, you should do HIT in a cool environment. A temperature between 65° and 70°F is best.

Illness and HIT

Question: Should I do the recommended exercises when I don't feel well?

Answer: No. HIT and illness both make heavy demands on your recovery ability. Illnesses can interfere with recovery from strenuous exercise, and strenuous exercise can aggravate some illnesses.

As a guideline, you should rest 1 day for every day you were sick before resuming your HIT plan. When you start exercising again, you should lower the intensity slightly for several workouts.

Influential Reading

Question: I have a nice collection of HIT books, including most of yours. Out of curiosity, what are some HIT books that you like?

Answer: First and foremost, Arthur Jones's *Nautilus Training Principles, Bulletin No. 1* (1970). If you've never studied this manual, you're in for a treat. You can read it on the Internet by going into the Web site www.MedXonline.com/Links and clicking into "Bulletin No. 1."

Second, I like Ken's Hutchins's *Super Slow: The Ultimate Exercise Protocol* (second edition, 1992). Ken and I grew up in the same hometown of Conroe, Texas. He worked for Nautilus for more than a dozen years and eventually started his own system of training based on repetition speed. Sometimes the chapters get technical, but if you're patient, you'll find lots of interesting guidelines discussed. You can order Hutchins's manual through www.Amazon.com.

Third, a recent compendium, which will cause you to scratch your head and think, is by Brian D. Johnston of Ontario, Canada, and is titled, *Exercise Science: Theory and Practice* (2003). Johnston's book is more than 1,000 pages and contains plenty of related bodybuilding and HIT materials. You can check it out on his Web site at www.IARTonline.ca.

There are a couple more books, which, if you have the time, are worth reviewing. *Building Strength and Stamina* (2003) by Wayne Westcott, Ph.D., covers HIT generally and Nautilus machines specifically. If you want a scientific, user-friendly resource concerning food and nutrition, get *Nutrition: Concepts and Controversies* (ninth edition, 2003) by Frances Sizer and Eleanor Whitney, Ph.D. Both of these books are available through www.Amazon.com.

Chapter 31

"I WOULD'VE TRAINED LESS": ARTHUR JONES LOOKS BACK

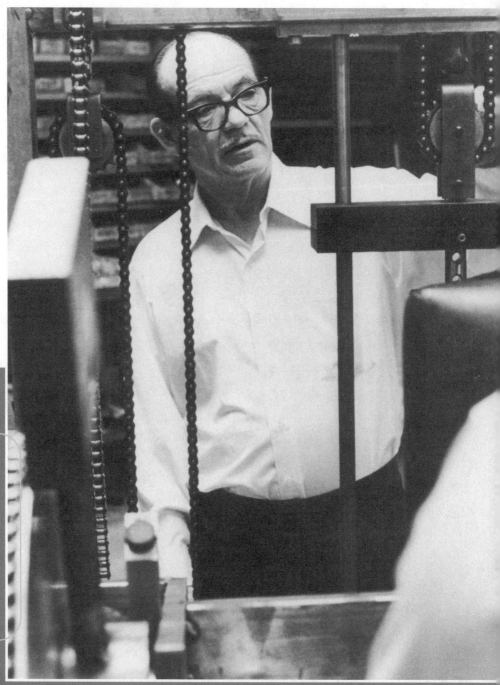

Arthur Jones has a history of studying cause and effect as they relate to lifting and muscle building. "If you are disappointed in your training results, before you apply anything else," Jones says, "try doing LESS exercise."

"HOW LONG DO you continue drinking a fluid if it doesn't quench your thirst? How long do you continue lifting weights if it doesn't produce bigger and stronger muscles?"

I've watched Arthur Jones study training for more than 30 years, examining what produces average versus excellent results. His analytical insights in the early 1970s provided the basic principles on which HIT was founded. His insights today are as crisp as when I first met him more than three decades ago—and they're fine-tuned with further experience.

That's why I want to close this book with a look at Jones's own training history.

Four Sets of 12 Exercises

Jones became interested in weight training when he was just 12. He also practiced gymnastics, which explains why chinups and dips were two of his favorite exercises. By 14, he was unusually strong and muscular.

He trained on and off over the next 15 years, because he was traveling the world and rarely had the necessary equipment. When he did train, he did three weekly workouts of four sets of 12 exercises.

Those workouts would bring him up to 172 pounds, where he'd inevitably hit a plateau. Additional work—more exercises, more sets—didn't do anything to lift him off the plateau. So, in disgust, he'd quit training for months or even years.

He would gradually lose muscle mass until he was down to 150 pounds. Then, when he his circumstances permitted, he'd start training again and inevitably get back up to 172. "Exactly 172 pounds, and not one ounce more," Jones said.

Finally, after several yo-yo journeys between 150

and 172 pounds, he decided to do something different—radically different. He cut his routine in half. Rather than four sets, he did just two sets of the 12 exercises.

Two Sets of 12 Exercises

"My body started growing, and quickly," Jones said. "It shocked even me." Within a few weeks, Jones was bigger and stronger than he'd ever been. He reasoned that the longer workouts hadn't allowed his body to get enough rest. In other words, he'd been overtraining.

When I visited him in Ocala on August 5, 2003, I asked him when he'd been at his biggest and strongest.

"It was in 1954 in Louisiana," he said. "I weighed 205 pounds with cold upper arms that measured $17\frac{1}{8}$ inches. And I was still doing two sets of 12 exercises, three times per week. That year, I could have entered and placed high in the Mr. America contest."

So I asked him what he would've done differently if he'd known then what he knows now.

"I would've trained less. Instead of 12 exercises, I would have reduced the number to 8. Instead of two sets, I would have performed only one set. Instead of training three times per week, I would have trained twice a week."

He doesn't know if he would've gotten bigger than his top weight of 205, but he's sure he would've gotten there faster.

Profit from Arthur Jones's Guidelines

If you were to sum up what Jones learned in 65 years of strength training, you could start with the following:

Be Realistic about Your Genetics

One of the last articles that Arthur Jones wrote for *IronMan* magazine (this was in the early 1990s) stressed the following to bodybuilders:

"Certain basic requirements for survival, things like food, water, air, and sleep, all of which must be provided by the environment, obviously have an influence on what we will be. But, given those basic requirements, what we actually will be is still primarily determined by genetics.

"Today, in this country alone, hundreds of millions of dollars are being literally stolen from people every year, stolen by convincing people that they can do things that are impossible. These things are possible for a few people, but impossible for most people."

Throughout this book, Arthur Jones and I have noted that most bodybuilders do not have the genetics to build muscular 18-inch arms and 50-inch chests—much less 20-inch arms and 54-inch chests. Such muscular achievements are not possible with HIT, high-volume training (HVT), massive amounts of drugs, or any other means. It's simply outside the realm of their physical capabilities.

(This is why you have to be at least a little skeptical when you read the claims and promises made in body-building magazines, whether those claims and promises refer to supplements, workout routines, or drugs.)

But at the same time, most serious bodybuilders can achieve a muscular pair of 16- to 17-inch upper arms, a 44- to 46-inch chest, and proportional shoulders, back, waist, and legs. And those are impressive dimensions.

As Chris Lund and I discussed in the introduction, competitive bodybuilding today is dominated by outrageous genetic freaks, who further complicate the situation by taking huge quantities of drugs. How these professionals exercise has little relationship to how the vast majority of bodybuilders, who are still interested in muscular size and strength, should train.

Apart from a very limited number of hard-core bodybuilders who are misguided enough to believe that they have a chance to compete against the genetic freaks, just about anybody else interested in bodybuilding can produce effective and efficient results from the application of the guidelines in this HIT book.

Understand clearly that with HIT and optimum rest, you can stimulate, develop, and maintain a great deal of muscular size and strength. But, in the assessment of your body's maximum capabilities, please try to be realistic.

• Two sets are better than four, and one set is better than two.

• Ten exercises are better than 12; for the most experienced lifters, 8 exercises are better than 10.

• For those experienced lifters, two workouts per week are better than three.

Sure, some athletes with the right genetics can grow to massive proportions on much higher exercise volume. Jones himself proved that. But these same athletes would have gotten even better results, and gotten them faster, if they'd trained less.

My advice: Don't assume you're an exception to these concepts. In fact, you'd be better off assuming that you're not.

It took Jones more than 30 years to learn that growth stimulation for a particular muscle requires only one set, properly performed. It took him another 20 years to understand that overall muscular growth accelerates from shorter routines and more rest days.

Make up your mind today that you're going to reach your full muscular potential in the most efficient manner: by training less.

Less and Harder

Jones challenged bodybuilders more than 30 years ago with the admonitions to train less and train harder. It took some of us a while, but those who successfully made the transition have never regretted it.

Training less and harder is the backbone of HIT. As you've seen throughout this book, HIT worked extremely well on the bodies of Casey Viator, Sergio Oliva, Mike Mentzer, Ray Mentzer, Boyer Coe, Scott Wilson, Dorian Yates, and, more recently, David Hudlow and Andy McCutcheon.

To make the transition, however, you may have to turn your back on the crowd. It requires guts to change directions in your training (or in anything else). Take charge—now.

Review . . .

Learn . . .

Plan . . .

Apply . . .

TRANSFORM.

Build solid muscle *fast* . . . with the new HIT!

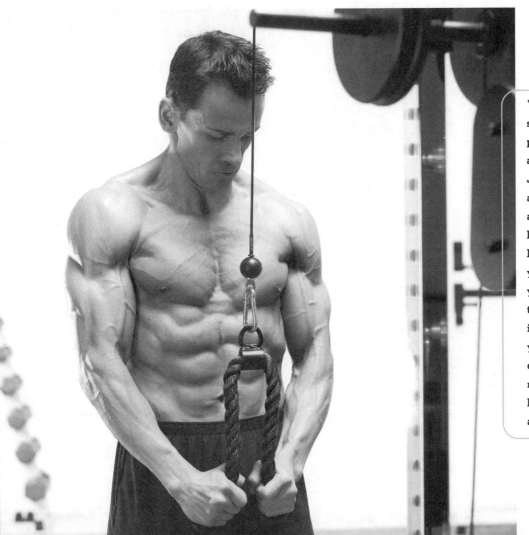

"Most bodybuilders seem to be willing to perform almost any amount of exercise," Jones said, "but they avoid anything actually approaching hard training." Don't let this happen to you. With practice, you can learn to train with great intensity. It's to your advantage to exercise smarter and more productively by working harder and briefer.

IT'S IMPORTANT TO keep an accurate record of your routines and workouts. Using a workout card like the one shown below will make the task easier. Simply fill in your exercises, as shown, in the left column. Then write in your resistance and number of repetitions (in good form) across from the exercise and under the date. When needed, add a plus sign (or an upward arrow) after the number of reps to indicate that the resistance was too light or a minus sign (or a downward arrow) to indicate that the weight was too heavy.

Turn the page for a blank workout card to photocopy and take to the gym.

NEW HIGH-INTENSITY TRAINING WORKOUT CARD							
EXERCISE	**Date**	10/10	10/12				
	Body weight	176	177				
1. Leg-Curl Machine		70 / 11	70 / 13 +				
2. Leg-Extension Machine		100 / 13 +	105 / 9				
3. Leg-Press Machine		180 / 6 −	170 / 9				
4. Straight-Arm Pullover with One Dumbbell		30 / 12 +	35 / 8				
5. Bench Press with Barbell		110 / 10	110 / 11				
6. Bent-Over Row with Barbell		80 / 10	80 / 13 +				
7. Overhead Press with Barbell		70 / 8	70 / 10				
8. Biceps Curl with Barbell		70 / 9	70 / 11				
9.							
10.							
11.							
12.							

NEW HIGH-INTENSITY TRAINING WORKOUT CARD							
EXERCISE	Date						
	Body weight						
1.							
2.							
3.							
4.							
5.							
6.							
7.							
8.							
9.							
10.							
11.							
12.							

Building solid, honest muscle in a safe, efficient manner—without the use of anabolic steroids—that's what HIT is about.

Boldface page references indicate photographs. <u>Underscored</u> references indicate boxed text.

T

U

V

Nutrition and Athletic Performance

Strength-Training Principles

Olympic Athletes Ask Questions about Exercise
   and Nutrition

How to Lose Body Fat

Soccer Fitness

How Your Muscles Work: Featuring Nautilus
   Training Equipment

Care and Conditioning of the Pitching Arm
   for Little League Baseball

Nutrition for Athletes: Myths and Truths

Conditioning for Football

Especially for Women

The Super-Fitness Handbook

The Nautilus Book

The Complete Encyclopedia of Weight Loss,
   Body Shaping, and Slenderizing

The Athletes Guide to Sports Medicine

Power Racquetball

Your Guide to Physical Fitness

The Nautilus Nutrition Book

The Nautilus Bodybuilding Book

The Darden Technique for Weight Loss

High-Intensity Bodybuilding

The Nautilus Woman

No More Fat

The Nautilus Advanced Bodybuilding Book

How to Look Terrific in a Bathing Suit

The Nautilus Handbook for Young Athletes

Super High-Intensity Bodybuilding

Massive Muscles in 10 Weeks

The Nautilus Diet

Big Arms in Six Weeks

100 High-Intensity Ways to Improve Your
   Bodybuilding

BIG: Bulkbuilding Instructional Guide

Bigger Muscles in 42 Days

The Six-Week Fat-to-Muscle Makeover

32 Days to a 32-Inch Waist

Hot Hips and Fabulous Thighs

Two Weeks to a Tighter Tummy

High-Intensity Strength Training

Grow

High-Intensity Home Training

The Positrim-Plus Diet Plan

Living Longer Stronger

Body Defining

Soft Steps to a Hard Body

A Flat Stomach ASAP

The Bowflex Body Plan

To contact Ellington Darden and explore the latest HIT developments, log on to www.DrDarden.com.

It's your last
HIT exercise.
Stay focused,
practice good form,
and make that final
repetition. You're
now ready to rest . . .
and *GROW!*